OPHTHALMOLOGY
MADE EASY

OPHTHALMOLOGY
MADE EASY

Michelle Attzs
BSc (Hons), MSc, MBBS, FRCOphth (Lon)
Attending Physician, Nemours Children's Health,
Jacksonville, Florida

and

Twishaa Sheth
BMedSci (Hons), BMBS (Hons), FRCOphth (Lon)
Specialist Registrar Ophthalmologist, East Suffolk
& North Essex NHS Foundation Trust

Scion

Scion Publishing Limited

The Old Hayloft, Vantage Business Park, Bloxham Road, Banbury OX16 9UX, UK

www.scionpublishing.com

Important Note from the Publisher

The information contained within this book was obtained by Scion Publishing Ltd from sources believed by us to be reliable. However, while every effort has been made to ensure its accuracy, no responsibility for loss or injury whatsoever occasioned to any person acting or refraining from action as a result of information contained herein can be accepted by the authors or publishers.

Readers are reminded that medicine is a constantly evolving science and while the authors and publishers have ensured that all dosages, applications and practices are based on current indications, there may be specific practices which differ between communities. You should always follow the guidelines laid down by the manufacturers of specific products and the relevant authorities in the country in which you are practising.

Although every effort has been made to ensure that all owners of copyright material have been acknowledged in this publication, we would be pleased to acknowledge in subsequent reprints or editions any omissions brought to our attention.

Registered names, trademarks, etc. used in this book, even when not marked as such, are not to be considered unprotected by law.

Cover design by Andrew Magee Design
Typeset by Evolution Design & Digital Ltd (Kent)
Printed in the UK

Last digit is the print number: 10 9 8 7 6 5 4 3 2

Contents

Foreword

Ophthalmology is a fascinating and wide-ranging high-volume outpatient specialty which has grown immensely due to recent advances in treatment and an ageing population demographic. This book provides a well-organized, practical and up-to-date approach to triage and diagnosis of a comprehensive range of common eye problems for a wide range of clinical practitioners.

The approach incorporates ophthalmic history-taking, examination and imaging methods, along with explanation of eye terminology, abbreviations, common eye medications and chapters on systemic infectious and inflammatory diseases. Important clinical concepts are highlighted in red. *Chapters 5* and *6* highlight important triage questions and symptoms which would be of particular interest to anyone doing clinical triage, such as GPs or GP trainees, nurses in A&E, eye emergency department, minor injury units or community optometrists doing minor eye conditions scheme or working in eye emergency departments. The book is superbly illustrated to support the clinical features of different eye conditions. Junior Ophthalmology trainees will find this book useful in the clinical setting for their patient care and knowing when to call for help or advice.

Ophthalmologists of all levels will find this text a useful teaching tool, particularly for providing a structure to teaching and simplifying complex topics and emphasizing important concepts for a non-specialist audience.

Miss Stella Hornby
MA (Cantab) MB BChir FRCOphth MD
Consultant Ophthalmologist specializing in
Primary Care Ophthalmology & Urgent Eye Care
Clinical Director of Ophthalmology
Oxford Eye Hospital, UK

Preface

Ophthalmology remains a bit of a dark art in the clinical world. It is barely covered in medical and clinical curriculums. Eye emergencies, however, can manifest themselves in any corner of the clinical environment, whether it be the GP surgery, outpatient clinic or A&E.

The first aim of this book is to build the confidence of non-ophthalmic clinicians on the initial assessment, management and onward referral to ophthalmology by discussing a) how to do the basics, b) what, and how, you can manage yourself, and c) when you might need to phone a friend. It will guide you through what to ask (and how to handle) that patient in your GP surgery with floaters, the patient on the ward with a red eye, or the patient in A&E with loss of vision.

The second aim is to give junior ophthalmologists the essential tips on how to manage some of the more common conditions they will encounter when they initially start their ophthalmology training. We appreciate that many books cover the foundations of ophthalmology superbly, in terms of anatomy, physiology and pathology, but we want this book to serve as an accessible reference guide.

It will be useful for medical students, foundation doctors, GPs, A&E doctors, junior ophthalmology specialty trainees, ophthalmic nurses and nurse practitioners, ophthalmic technicians or anyone looking to refresh their knowledge of diagnosis, management and referral to ophthalmology.

This is the book we wish we had had as medical students and juniors.

Michelle Attzs
Twishaa Sheth

About the authors

Michelle Attzs

Michelle is a post CCT fellow of the Royal College of Ophthalmologists, who completed her training with the East Midlands Deanery, which includes Nottingham University Hospitals NHS Trust where she was awarded Trainee of the Year 2019. She has completed two prestigious fellowships in paediatric ophthalmology and strabismus at Wilmer Eye Institute, Johns Hopkins and Bascom Palmer Eye Institute, University of Miami. Throughout her career, Michelle has been dedicated to teaching peers both within and outside the field of ophthalmology, and her ultimate goal is to equip learners with the tools to appreciate and understand the structure, function and disease of the eye. Michelle is currently an Attending Physician at Nemours Children's Health, Jacksonville, Florida.

Twishaa Sheth

Twishaa is a Specialist Registrar Ophthalmologist at East Suffolk & North Essex NHS Foundation Trust in the East of England Deanery; this includes Cambridge University Hospitals where she was awarded the Marie Comer Ophthalmology Prize. She was awarded the Harcourt Gold Medal in 2023 for the highest mark achieved in the final Fellowship of the Royal College of Ophthalmologists Exit Examinations on her first attempt. She is now a formal examiner for the Royal College of Ophthalmologists. She is currently also undertaking an MSc at the University of Oxford. She has a heartfelt passion for teaching ophthalmology and making it accessible to those who are new to the subject.

Contributors

The completion of this book would not have been possible without the contribution to each chapter by ophthalmologists and allied ophthalmology staff around the world.

Mr Giorgio Albanese, MD, FEBO
Consultant, Oculoplastics and Orbit
Nottingham University Hospitals NHS Trust, UK

Miss Lana Faraj, MD, MSc, PhD, FRCOphth
Consultant, Cornea and Anterior Segment
University Hospitals of Derby and Burton NHS Foundation Trust, UK

Dr Cherie Fathy, MD MPH
Medical Officer, Food and Drug Administration
Silver Spring, MD, USA

Dr Karishma Habbu, MD
Attending Physician, Advanced Eye Care
Baltimore, MD, USA

Miss Delicia Jayakumar, MBBS, DO, MRCOphth, FRCOphth
Specialty Doctor in Ophthalmology
Sherwood Forest Hospitals NHS Foundation Trust, UK

Mr Z HH Lin, FRCOphth, FEBO, FICO, PGCert (Cantab)
Consultant, Oculoplastic & Lacrimal Surgery, Medical Law
East Suffolk and North Essex NHS Foundation Trust, UK

Miss Archana Pradeep, MBBS, MD, FRCOphth, PGCert Genomic Medicine
Consultant, Uveitis and Inflammatory Eye Diseases
Queen's Medical Centre, Nottingham University Hospitals NHS Trust, UK

Dr Cody Richardson, MD
Assistant Professor, Paediatric Ophthalmology and Adult Strabismus
Wilmer Eye Institute, Johns Hopkins Hospital, Baltimore, MD, USA

Charlotte Tibi, CO
Senior Certified Orthoptist, Department of Paediatric Ophthalmology and Strabismus
Bascom Palmer Eye Institute, University of Miami, Miami, FL, USA

Dr Jonathan Tijerina, MD, MA
Ophthalmology Trainee, Bascom Palmer Eye Institute
University of Miami, Miami, FL, USA

Miss Olayinka Williams, BSc (Hons), MBBS, FRCOphth
Post CCT Fellow, Moorfields Eye Hospital, London, UK

Nadia Wong, BA, COMT, CDOS, ROUB
Certified Ophthalmic Technician, Department of Echography
Wilmer Eye Institute, Johns Hopkins Hospital, Baltimore, MD, USA

How to use this book

Chapters 1 and *2* give a primer on how to take a basic eye history and examine an eye without any specialist equipment, so that outside of the ophthalmology department, you can still make safe diagnoses and referrals. *Chapters 3* and *4* provide a glossary of common ophthalmic terminology and medication, which will be a useful reference when reviewing those ophthalmology letters. For triaging eye complaints, use *Chapters 5* and *6* to 'sort the symptoms' and help decide how soon you need to refer the patient or, if you are the one working in ophthalmology, when to accept them.

Chapters 7 to *16* offer a system-based approach to each part of the eye. They highlight common and important conditions whilst describing how to assess, investigate, manage and refer if needed, and what to do if you're the first ophthalmic clinician seeing the patient. *Chapters 17* to *20* describe common ophthalmic investigations, and *Chapters 21* and *22* cover ophthalmic manifestations of systemic disease.

Throughout the book, symbols are used to highlight what parts of assessment and management are relevant to non-ophthalmic and ophthalmic clinicians.

 This symbol indicates history, examination, investigations or management that could or should be undertaken in a non-ophthalmology setting. Such sections are aimed at non-ophthalmic clinicians.

 This symbol indicates history, examination, investigations or management that could or should be undertaken by an ophthalmologist or clinician working in an ophthalmology department. Sections marked thus are aimed at junior ophthalmology specialty trainees, ophthalmic nurses and nurse practitioners.

CLINICAL CONTEXT TIPS

These boxes will help to add 'the bigger picture' or further your understanding of the conditions described.

RED FLAG

These boxes highlight important clinical concepts that should never be missed.

Bold text highlights key referral tips. Red text highlights sight- or life-threatening pathology.

Image acknowledgements

The majority of the images included in the book are from our personal collections and from the collections of the contributors. For other images, we have indicated their source, and we thank the publishers and authors for granting permission.

General abbreviations

For specific abbreviations used in an ophthalmology report, see *Chapter 3*.

A&E	Accident and Emergency	GI	gastrointestinal
ACD	anterior chamber depth	GP	general practitioner
ACE	angiotensin-converting enzyme	GPA	granulomatosis with polyangiitis
ANA	antinuclear antibodies	HIV	human immunodeficiency virus
ARN	acute retinal necrosis	HSV	herpes simplex virus
BG	blood glucose	ICP	intracranial pressure
BP	blood pressure	IOL	intraocular lens
CCF	carotid-cavernous fistula	LPS	levator palpebrae superioris
CN	cranial nerve	MDT	multidisciplinary team
CNP	cranial nerve palsy	MRI	magnetic resonance imaging
COPD	chronic obstructive pulmonary disease	MuSK	muscle-specific kinase
		NAI	non-accidental injury
CPEO	chronic progressive external ophthalmoplegia	NSAID	non-steroidal anti-inflammatory drug
CRP	C-reactive protein	PCR	polymerase chain reaction
CSF	cerebrospinal fluid	PMR	polymyalgia rheumatica
CSNB	congenital stationary night blindness	PUK	peripheral ulcerative keratitis
		RA	rheumatoid arthritis
CT	computed tomography	RF	rheumatoid factor
DED	dry eye disease	RPE	retinal pigment epithelium
DR	diabetic retinopathy	RVO	retinal vein occlusion
DVLA	Driver and Vehicle Licensing Agency	SJS	Stevens–Johnson syndrome
		TED	thyroid eye disease
ECG	electrocardiogram	TIA	transient ischaemic attack
ENT	ear, nose and throat	TSH	thyroid-stimulating hormone
ESR	erythrocyte sedimentation rate	VFD	visual field defect
FBC	full blood count	VZV	varicella zoster virus

Chapter 1
Basic ophthalmic history

1.1 Introduction

Medical school traditionally prepares you very well for medical and surgical history-taking. During your foundation years and beyond you come to develop a good, structured approach to history-taking for most presenting complaints.

However, when it comes to the eye, it can be very tempting as a knee-jerk reaction to 'refer to ophthalmology' any patient with an ocular complaint.

Although your local or senior ophthalmologist is usually more than happy to be approached and provide advice, many problems can be differentiated (or at least narrowed down) by a good history alone. So, regardless of whether you are a general practitioner (GP), medical student, nurse practitioner or junior doctor, you should ensure that you can take a good ophthalmology history, and doing so will help to provide a comprehensive but focused referral if you do need to pick up the phone.

We are taught traditionally to ask open questions when history-taking and, although this approach has its merits, ocular complaints are dealt with better if the history involves slightly more structure and direct questioning (especially in busy Accident and Emergency (A&E) settings), as explained below.

Please note: any urgent life- or sight-threatening conditions have been highlighted in red text below.

1.2 History of presenting complaint

Generally, the presenting complaints of the eye conditions you are likely to come across commonly can be divided into three broad categories.

How the eye is seeing

- **Not being able to see:**
  - either part or all of the visual field
  - either persistent or transient loss of vision
  - blurring
  - complete loss of vision
  - distortion.
- **Seeing new things:**
  - flashes
  - floaters
  - patterns
  - haloes
  - glare
  - double vision
  - hallucinations.

CLINICAL CONTEXT TIPS

Not being able to see
- Subjective visual field deficit should also be characterized as to which part of the field is missing:
  - central scotomas indicate macular or optic nerve pathology
  - peripheral vision loss can come from branch vascular occlusions or retinal detachments
  - a homonymous (affecting the same part of the visual field of each eye – right visual field or left visual field) defect indicates neurological aetiology.
- Transient vision loss should trigger thoughts of amaurosis fugax, although it can also happen in pigment dispersion syndrome and as a result of raised intracranial pressure.
- Complete, acute loss of vision could represent vascular pathology such as retinal artery or vein occlusions, ischaemic optic neuropathy, vitreous haemorrhage or retinal detachment.
- Distortion indicates macular pathology such as macular oedema, epiretinal membrane, macular holes or age-related macular degeneration.

Seeing new things
- Flashes and floaters generally indicate a vitreoretinal interface cause.
- Patterns, especially if seen bilaterally, point more towards a neurological cause or migraine.
- Haloes can be a sign of corneal oedema from raised intraocular pressure, for instance from acute angle closure.
- Glare is a common complaint from symptomatic cataract.
- Double vision should be characterized as either binocular (present with both eyes open but goes away when you close either eye) or monocular (only present in one eye, i.e. still present in that eye when you close the other).
- Hallucinations can be part of Charles Bonnet syndrome, which can occur in conditions causing severe visual loss. Patients rarely volunteer that they are experiencing them, so they should be asked about specifically if suspected.

How the eye looks
- Red eye
  - partly red / sectoral rednes
  - diffusely red
- Discharge
  - watery
  - 'just crusting'
  - purulent
- Lid abnormalities – swelling, lumps, drooping
- Eye turning in/out/up/down

How the eye looks
- Red eye:
  - circumlimbal ➜ corneal or uveal pathology
  - sectoral ➜ episcleritis, inflamed pinguecula or pterygium
- Discharge:
  - watery ➜ allergic and viral aetiology
  - purulent ➜ bacterial aetiology
- Crusting (especially in the mornings) ➜ blepharitis

How the eye feels
- Itchy
- Gritty or dry
- Foreign body sensation
- Discomfort
- Pain
- Photosensitivity.

- An itchy eye (i.e. the feeling of wanting to rub it) can indicate hypersensitivity or allergic conjunctivitis.
- A gritty or uncomfortable eye can indicate ocular surface problems (e.g. dry eyes) and discomfort is associated with episcleritis.
- A foreign body sensation or a sharp, searing pain which makes it difficult to open the eyes points towards corneal pathology (e.g. an abrasion, foreign body or keratitis).
- Photosensitivity can occur in corneal or uveal pathology (e.g. acute anterior uveitis).

This may sound obvious, but it is vital to narrow down in which eye the symptoms are being experienced. Patients with homonymous hemianopia, for instance, may attribute their symptoms to their 'right eye' as opposed to 'the right field of both eyes'. It is also always important to check that their 'good' eye is indeed non-symptomatic.

It is also crucial to assess the timing of the symptoms because this can often help you either:
- triage the referral
- assess your urgency in referring to ophthalmology.

As a general rule, an acute loss of vision (e.g. 2 hours ago) should be seen urgently, whereas loss of vision over a period of months could be referred routinely.

Once you have filtered down the patient's core presenting symptoms, the onset of each symptom, their nature, severity and course can be assessed much as you would with a medical history.

1.3 Systems review

System review features that may be relevant in your history are:

1.3.1 Possible giant cell arteritis (GCA)

- Headache (temporal)
- Scalp tenderness
- Jaw or tongue claudication
- Polymyalgia rheumatica (PMR) symptoms: neck or shoulder girdle pain, hip pain
- Systemic malaise: anorexia, weight loss or fever
- Neurological symptoms: gait / speech / swallow.

1.3.2 Red eye

- Recent trauma
- Rashes or cold sores
- Gastrointestinal (GI), genito-urinary or musculoskeletal symptoms
- Upper respiratory tract infections
- Subconjunctival haemorrhage risk factors: recent straining / constipation, coughing, trauma, use of blood thinners.

1.3.3 Loss of vision

- Neurological symptoms: gait / speech / swallow suggestive of a stroke (although loss of vision, and in particular, loss of field of vision may be the only symptom a patient who has suffered a stroke has).

1.3.4 Possible acute angle closure

- Nausea, vomiting
- Headaches.

1.3.5 Possible raised intracranial pressure

- Pulsatile tinnitus
- Vomiting
- Gait/speech difficulties.

1.4 Background history

This is as relevant in ophthalmology as it is in any other specialty, with its own special section for past ocular history. It is important to document this regardless of whether the initial consultation is in general practice, in triage, in A&E, or in the ophthalmology department, because it not only guides your assessment but streamlines your referral.

1.4.1 Past ocular history

- Previous ocular diagnoses; for instance, similar symptoms in a patient with a history of recurrent acute anterior uveitis is likely to represent a flare
- Previous ocular trauma
- Previous ocular surgery (including laser – ask specifically because patients can forget to mention it!)
- Previous contact lens wear
- Amblyopia; ask *"has this eye been weaker since childhood?"*
  - it's a common misconception that a 'lazy eye' is a squint or turn in the eye
  - amblyopia actually refers to abnormal visual development in early life (i.e. 0–8 years of age) causing reduced vision.

1.4.2 Past medical history

Past medical history is not only relevant in formulating a differential diagnosis (as some systemic conditions have ophthalmic associations or require ophthalmic screening for their treatment), but it is also important because certain conditions preclude treatment given for ophthalmic conditions. Some examples of associations (or pertinent negatives – it is important to document these) include:

- Red eye: ask about atopy or rheumatological conditions
- Loss of vision: ask about hypertension, diabetes, hyperlipidaemia, neurological diagnoses
- Floaters: ask about diabetes or systemic connective tissue disease
- Headache: ask about neurological diagnoses or PMR
- Glaucoma clinic: ask about asthma, chronic obstructive pulmonary disease (COPD), or sickle cell disease (these can be contraindications to certain glaucoma medications).

1.4.3 Drug history

Ensure that you document:

- Allergies
- Any medication recently started which might act as a trigger for ophthalmic conditions, for example:
  - anticholinergics which may trigger acute angle closure
  - any corticosteroid use which can trigger central serous retinopathy.

1.4.4 Family history

Check close family contacts for infective symptoms (e.g. in viral conjunctivitis), general ocular family history (e.g. glaucoma, retinal detachments, strabismus) and genetic systemic / ophthalmic conditions.

1.4.5 Social history

This is vital in ophthalmology and so be sure to include:

- Activities of daily living: how does the patient's eye condition affect how they live their life?

- Smoking / alcohol status: this is relevant in certain ophthalmic diagnoses
- Driving status: ask the patient directly if they are driving, as you are duty bound to advise them to inform the Driver and Vehicle Licensing Agency (DVLA) in the UK, should they not reach the driving vision standards, or be diagnosed with certain conditions.

To help focus your history even further, please see *Chapter 5* (*Focusing your history: sorting the symptoms*).

Chapter 2
Basic ophthalmic anatomy and examination

2.1 Introduction

The eye is a complex structure with distinct compartments. Although the adnexal (orbit and eyelids) and the anterior segment (conjunctiva, cornea, iris and lens) are visible to the naked eye, a closer assessment of the lens, iridocorneal angle, vitreous and fundus calls for a more in-depth examination with the slit lamp or ophthalmoscope. In pre-ophthalmology settings such as primary care and A&E, there is often no slit lamp available, nor anyone trained to use it effectively. With this in mind, this chapter will not only cover the anatomy of the orbital and ocular structures, but will also provide clinical context tips on how to examine some structures of the eye in a pre-ophthalmology setting, without the use of a slit lamp or any other specialist equipment. However, we will start by illustrating how to assess for visual function.

2.2 Assessment of visual function

Vision, colour vision and visual field provide information about visual function, and changes to them (along with a thorough history; see *Chapter* 1) can guide a clinician to the underlying cause of the patient's presentation.

A Snellen chart (*Appendix 1*) and a near vision reading chart (*Appendix 2*) are the most formal ways of documenting distant and near visual acuity in children over the age of 3 and adults, whilst a colour vision chart (also known as an Ishihara chart) allows formal documentation of colour vision. Non-ophthalmic clinical areas may or may not have these tools, so there are other techniques (and more recently, mobile phone Snellen apps) to help decipher if there is any asymmetry in vision between the patient's eyes:
- Check if the patient wears glasses or contact lens for distance or near vision (or both)
- Ask them to wear their glasses or contacts if available
- Ask the patient to cover one eye
- Distance vision:
  - either stand in front of the patient at a distance of approximately 6 metres and ask them to recall how many fingers you are holding up, or
  - ask the patient to read a poster/screen at a similar distance
- Near vision:
  - ask the patient to read the text on a leaflet or your name on your ID badge
- Colour vision:
  - ask the patient to look at a red object
- Test the opposite eye
- Document:

    ○ testing done monocularly (each eye separately) or binocularly (both eyes open)
    ○ testing done with or without glasses or contact lens
    ○ any asymmetry in responses between the two eyes.

2.3 Orbit

The orbit is a complex of seven bony structures: ethmoid, frontal, lacrimal, maxillary, palatine, sphenoid and zygomatic (*Figure 2.1*). Its embryological origin is a combination of the neural crest, mesoderm and ectoderm. The function of the orbit is to protect the contents of the orbit, and provide sufficient space for ocular movement, although there is a relatively small amount of space between the orbital walls and the globe. The sphenoid and maxillary bones contain foramina (or canals) which also permit the passage of nerves from the eye to the brain.

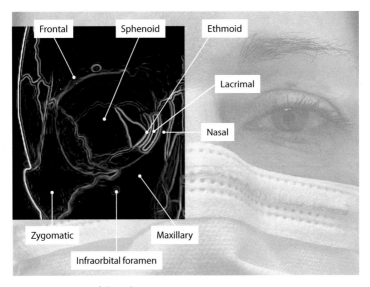

Figure 2.1 Bones of the orbit.

CLINICAL CONTEXT TIPS

How to examine the orbit
CT and MRI imaging is very useful in diagnosis of orbital pathology; examination of the orbit is essential as part of the work-up. Inspection of the periorbital and orbital areas will identify:
- Eyelid swelling
- Eyelid bruising
- Change in eyelid position
- Skin discolouration

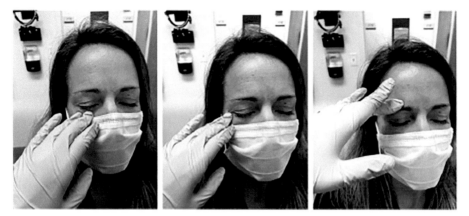

Figure 2.2 Palpation technique for the orbital rim (left to right: maxilla, zygoma and frontal bone).

- Obvious mass lesions
- Globe displacement (forward, i.e. proptosis, vertical / horizontal, i.e. dystopia, backward, i.e. enophthalmos; compare to the contralateral eye)
- Pulsation of the globe.

Palpation of the bony orbital rim (*Figure 2.2*) is useful for identifying:
- Discontinuity of the orbital rim
- Emphysema (air) under the subcutaneous tissue of the orbit (felt as crepitus / crackling on palpation of the orbital rim)
- Foreign bodies
- Masses.

Further components of examination of the orbit include:
- Place palm over closed eyelids and feel for a vibration whilst palpating the radial pulse
- Gently press over closed eyelid with two fingers and check for resistance to retropulsion
- Ask the patient to bend forward and observe if any proptosis gets worse
- Document:
  - visual acuity and colour vision (see *Section 2.2*)
  - changes in visual field (see *Section 14.2*)
  - eye movements (see *Section 2.4.5*)
  - pupillary responses (see *Figure 2.20*)
- Assess lid closure
- Bell's phenomenon:
  - can you see any of the sclera or cornea with forced lid closure whilst you try to open the lids?
- Assess the conjunctiva for redness and cornea for any opacity.

2.4 Adnexal structures

2.4.1 Eyelids

The eyelids serve to protect the globe and the orbital contents. During embryonic development, the eyelids form from contributions between the mesenchyme and the surface ectoderm. The blink mechanism facilitates the spread of tears over the ocular surface. The height of the upper lid is more than that of the lower lid. The resting position of the upper eyelid is 1–2 mm below the superior corneoscleral limbus, whilst that of the lower eyelid is at the inferior corneoscleral limbus. *Section 8.3* discusses the measurements required when assessing pathology of the eyelids, such as ptosis.

Moving from anterior to posterior (*Figure 2.3*), the layers of the eyelids comprise:
- Skin (anterior lamella)
  - eyelashes
  - sebaceous glands (which can give rise to cyst of Zeis; see *Section 8.6.1*)
  - sweat glands (which can give rise to the cyst of Moll; see *Section 8.6.1*)
- Subcutaneous connective tissue (anterior lamella)
- Orbicularis oculi muscle (anterior lamella)
  - involved in blinking and facial expression
  - innervated by the facial nerve (cranial nerve (CN) VII)
  - split into orbital and palpebral segments
  - the most superficial aspect of the palpebral segment becomes the Riolan muscle, which corresponds to the grey line (*Figure 2.4*) which separates the lid into anterior and posterior lamella (layers)
- Orbital septum
  - extension of the periosteum from the superior orbital rim
  - important in distinguishing between preseptal and orbital cellulitis (see *Section 7.4.2*)
- Upper eyelid muscle: levator palpebrae superioris (LPS) muscle
  - elevates and retracts the upper eyelid
  - combines with the superior rectus to form the Whitnall ligament, at which the LPS divides into the levator aponeurosis and the superior (Müller) muscle
  - the insertion of the LPS/Müller muscle into the superior aspect of the tarsal plate forms the upper eyelid crease
  - innervated by the superior division oculomotor nerve (CN III)
- Lower eyelid muscle: inferior tarsal muscle
  - extends from the inferior tarsal plate and the inferior fornix
  - maintains the position of the lower eyelid
  - connects to the inferior rectus via the lower lid retractors, which means the downward movement of the lower eyelids occurs with downward gaze
- Tarsal plate (posterior lamella)
  - a thickened extension of the orbital septum
  - measures 10mm on the upper eyelid and 5mm on the lower eyelid
  - contains the meibomian glands, which supply the oil layer of the tear film (see *Section 2.4*)

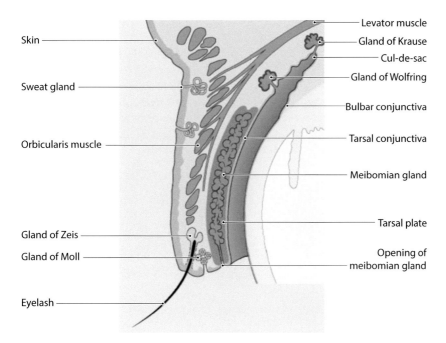

Skin

Sweat gland

Orbicularis muscle

Gland of Zeis

Gland of Moll

Eyelash

Levator muscle

Gland of Krause

Cul-de-sac

Gland of Wolfring

Bulbar conjunctiva

Tarsal conjunctiva

Meibomian gland

Tarsal plate

Opening of meibomian gland

Figure 2.3 Cross-section of upper eyelid.

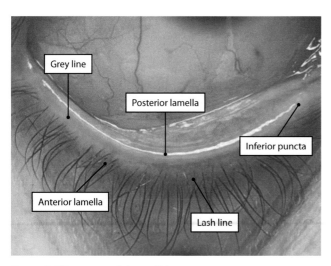

Grey line

Posterior lamella

Inferior puncta

Anterior lamella

Lash line

Figure 2.4 Structures of the eyelid.

- Conjunctiva (posterior lamella)
  - mucous membrane
  - stratified squamous epithelium
  - contains goblet cells which produce the mucin layer of the tear film (see *Section 2.4*).

11

Eyelids have a dual arterial supply from the external carotid artery system (via the facial and angular artery supplying the medial eyelid, and the temporal artery supplying the lateral eyelid) and internal carotid artery system (supplying the supraorbital and lacrimal arteries). This blood supply also feeds the superior and inferior marginal, and superior peripheral arterial arcades of the eyelids. There is also a dual venous drainage with a pretarsal, or superficial, drainage into the internal and external jugular veins, and a post-tarsal, or deep, drainage into the cavernous sinus. The medial eyelid drains into the submandibular lymph nodes, whilst the lateral eyelid drains into the preauricular lymph nodes (often tender in viral conjunctivitis).

CLINICAL CONTEXT TIPS

How to examine the eyelids
- Observe eyelids for:
  - discharge
  - swelling
  - redness
  - lumps or bumps
  - position:
    - is one eyelid lower than the other?
    - is the eyelid turning in or out?

2.4.2 Conjunctival sac

The conjunctival sac is an anatomical space between the palpebral and bulbar conjunctiva (see *Figure 2.10*). Aside from allowing a reservoir for tears and eye drops, the conjunctival sac serves to allow the eyelids to move smoothly over the eye.

CLINICAL CONTEXT TIPS

How to examine the conjunctival sac
Ask the patient to look up, and gently pull down the lower lid to view the inferior fornix (the pocket between the bulbar conjunctiva over the globe, and palpebral conjunctiva on the inside of the eyelid), observing for a foreign body, or shallowing / symblepharon which occurs in ocular cicatricial pemphigoid.

2.4.3 Tear production

There is basal and reflex production of tears.

Basal production is performed by the meibomian glands, the glands and goblet cells of the conjunctiva and the lacrimal gland, whilst only the lacrimal gland is involved in reflex production.

The tear film provides moisture and nutrition to the conjunctiva and cornea, and a clear refractive surface to the cornea. It consists of three layers:
- Phospholipid (oil, outer) layer
  - produced by the meibomian glands of the eyelids
  - increases the surface tension of the tear film to prevent premature evaporation
- Aqueous (water, middle) layer (the most abundant layer)
  - produced by the lacrimal and accessory glands (glands of Krause and Wolfring) of the conjunctiva
  - provides moisture and nutrients to the cornea and conjunctiva
- Mucin (protein, inner) layer
  - produced by the conjunctival goblet cells
  - facilitates the adherence of the hydrophilic tear film to the hydrophobic cornea epithelium.

The lacrimal gland is an exocrine gland situated in the superotemporal orbit (see *Figures 2.5* and *2.6*). It forms from the neural crest during embryonic development. It is a bilobar gland, with a larger orbital lobe and a small palpebral lobe, separated by the levator palpebrae superioris aponeurosis. It receives its blood supply from the internal carotid artery system via the ophthalmic and lacrimal artery, and its venous drainage is into the cavernous sinus via the superior ophthalmic vein. The parasympathetic system, via the lacrimal nerve (small branch of the ophthalmic branch of the trigeminal nerve), increases secretion from the lacrimal gland.

2.4.4 Nasolacrimal system

The nasolacrimal system (*Figure 2.5*) comprises the following components:
- Superior (upper) and inferior (lower) puncta
- Superior and inferior canaliculi, which usually fuse to become the common canaliculus (in 90% of individuals)
- The lacrimal sac, which is 12mm long, and sits in the lacrimal fossa
- The nasolacrimal duct, which is 18mm long, which opens in the inferior meatus in the nose.

Tears are excreted with the assistance of the blink mechanism, which provides a pumping action to drive tears into the lacrimal sac and down the nasolacrimal duct.

CLINICAL CONTEXT TIPS

How to examine the lacrimal gland and the lacrimal sac
An enlarged lacrimal gland can be visualized with the naked eye by lifting the upper eyelid and asking the patient to look down and far nasally (*Figure 2.6A*).

If lacrimal sac pathology is suspected, pressing just lateral to the medial canthus and observing any fluctuance / reflux suggests nasolacrimal duct obstruction (*Figure 2.6B*).

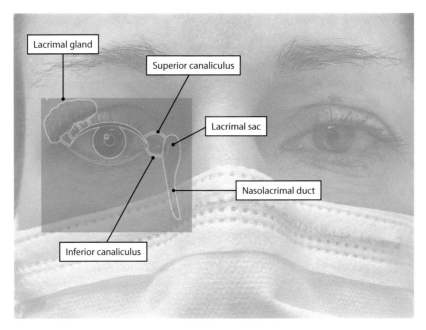

Figure 2.5 Lacrimal gland and nasolacrimal system.

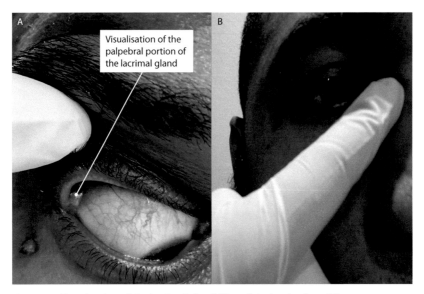

Figure 2.6 Examination of the lacrimal gland (A) and the lacrimal sac (B).

2.4.5 Extraocular muscles

There are six extraocular muscles (EOMs) (*Figure 2.7*) involved in the nine cardinal movements of the eye. During embryonic development they are formed from the mesodermal mesenchyme. *Table 2.1* describes the EOMs, including their origins, insertions and nerve supplies.

Table 2.1 Origins, insertions and nerve supply of the extraocular muscles

Muscle	Origin	Insertion	Nerve supply
Medial rectus (MR)	Annulus of Zinn	5.5mm from limbus	Oculomotor (CN III)
Lateral rectus (LR)	Annulus of Zinn	7.0mm from limbus	Abducens (CN VI)
Superior rectus (SR)	Annulus of Zinn	7.5mm from limbus	Oculomotor (CN III)
Inferior rectus (IR)	Annulus of Zinn	6.5mm from limbus	Oculomotor (CN III)
Superior oblique (SO)	Sphenoid bone	Posterior superotemporal, inferior to SR	Trochlear (CN IV)
Inferior oblique (IO)	Orbital floor	Posterior temporal, inferior to LR	Oculomotor (CN III)

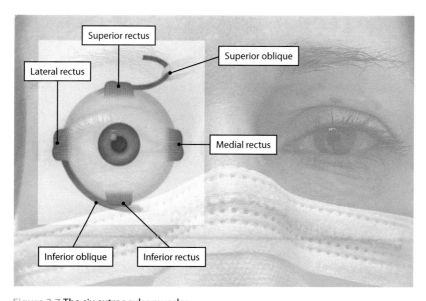

Figure 2.7 The six extraocular muscles.

Eye movements are either monocular or binocular. Monocular movements are known as ductions (*Table 2.2*), and binocular movements are versions (*Figure 2.8*).

Two laws govern the actions of the EOM:

- Hering's law of equal innervation – innervation to yoke muscles is equal, i.e. two muscles that are responsible for the movement of the eye in a particular direction of gaze receive equal innervation, e.g. lateral rectus of right eye and medial rectus of left eye for right horizontal gaze
- Sherrington's law – innervation to a muscle is accompanied by decreased innervation of its antagonist muscles, e.g. increased innervation to lateral rectus of right eye with decreased innervation to the medial rectus of the right eye for right horizontal gaze.

The cardinal movements of the eye include primary position, right and left gaze, straight up, up and left, up and right, straight down, down and left, and down and right. *Figure 2.7* illustrates the muscles involved with each eye position.

Table 2.2 Actions of the extraocular muscles

EOM	Primary	Secondary	Tertiary
Medial rectus	Adduction	–	–
Lateral rectus	Abduction	–	–
Superior rectus	Elevation	Intorsion	Adduction
Inferior rectus	Depression	Extorsion	Adduction
Superior oblique	Intorsion	Depression	Abduction
Inferior oblique	Extorsion	Elevation	Abduction

Each EOM obtains its blood supply from branches of the ophthalmic artery (a branch of the internal carotid artery). A fascial layer called the Tenon's capsule lies between the conjunctiva and the EOM, and encapsulates each EOM.

CLINICAL CONTEXT TIPS

How to assess ocular motility
The ability of a patient to move their eyes smoothly can be assessed by asking the patient to *"follow the tip of my pen without moving your head"* (*Figure 2.9*). This is repeated for all nine positions of gaze, assessing each extraocular muscle in turn (see *Figure 2.8*).

2.5 Conjunctiva and cornea

2.5.1 Conjunctiva

The anatomy of the conjunctiva was described in *Section 2.4.1*. There are three parts to the conjunctival complex of the eye:

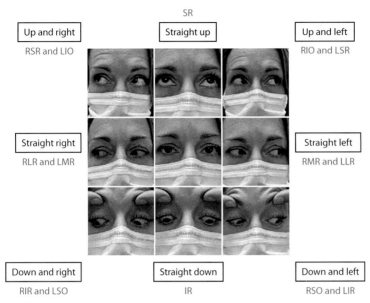

Figure 2.8 The nine cardinal eye positions and the muscles that control them.
LIO, left inferior oblique; LIR, left inferior rectus; LLR, left lateral rectus; LMR, left medial rectus; LSO, left superior oblique; LSR, left superior rectus; RIO, right inferior oblique; RIR, right inferior rectus; RLR, right lateral rectus; RMR, right medial rectus; RSO, right superior oblique; RSR, right superior rectus, SR, superior rectus, IR, inferior rectus.

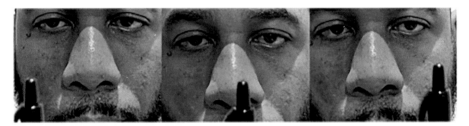

Figure 2.9 Examination of eye movement, asking the patient to follow the tip of the pen without moving their head.

- Palpebral conjunctiva lines the posterior layer of the eyelids (seen as the pink inner lining of the eyelid, when you pull the lower eyelid down)
- Bulbar conjunctiva lines the globe (seen as the white of the eye)
- Forniceal (superior and inferior) conjunctiva is the loose mobile junction between the palpebral and bulbar parts (*Figure 2.10*).

2.5.2 Cornea

The cornea is an avascular, transparent structure which contributes to the refractive (focusing) power of the eye; approximately two-thirds of the refractive power of the eye

17

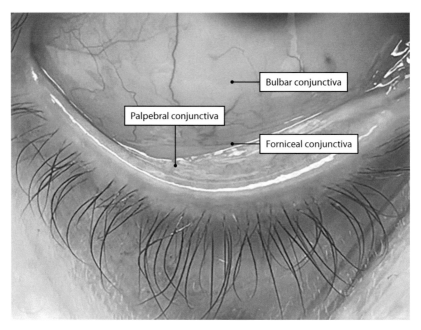

Figure 2.10 The locations of the bulbar, palpebral and forniceal conjunctiva.

comes from the cornea. It comprises five layers, all with a unique histopathological make-up (*Figure 2.11*). The cornea is also unique in that each layer has a different embryological origin:

- The epithelium and the Bowman's layer form from the surface ectodermal cells
- The stroma is formed from the mesoderm
- The endothelium and Descemet's membrane form from the neural crest cells.

On average, the adult cornea has a diameter of 11–12mm horizontally, with a centrally thinner section (approximately 535µm), and a thicker periphery (approximately 660µm). It has an elliptical shape anteriorly (i.e. it is longer in the horizontal plane compared to the vertical plane), and a circular shape posteriorly. It is supplied by the nasociliary nerves and the long ciliary nerves which originate from the ophthalmic division of the trigeminal nerve.

CLINICAL CONTEXT TIPS

How to examine the cornea

Assessment of the corneal surface can readily be done with a pen torch; however, a more in-depth look at its structure requires a slit lamp. Observe the cornea:

- Is it clear (iris details clearly visible) or cloudy?
- If fluorescein 2% and the blue cobalt light (*Figure 2.12*) on a pen torch, or indirect ophthalmoscope is available, observe for epithelial defects, foreign bodies or lacerations.

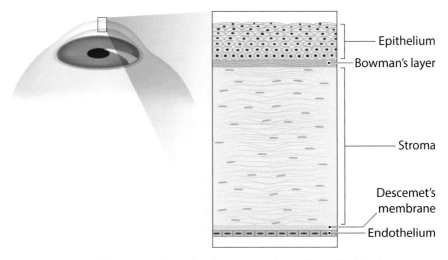

Figure 2.11 Layers of the cornea. Adapted with permission from Alila Medical Media.

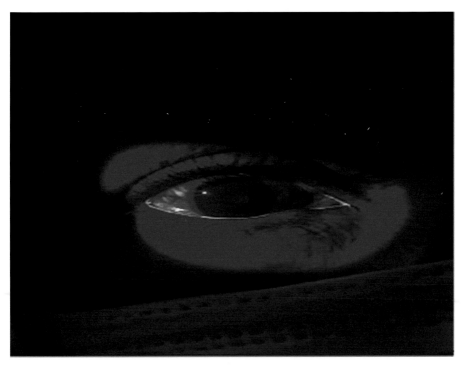

Figure 2.12 Use of fluorescein 2% and a blue cobalt light to assess the integrity of the ocular surface. Insert a drop of fluorescein into the eye, then shine the cobalt blue light over the eye (in dim room light for better visualization). Any discrete areas of 'bright green' uptake represent corneal epithelial defects, such as from a scratch, ulcer or foreign body. In this image, there is no fluorescein uptake on the cornea, suggesting the integrity of the cornea is normal.

2.6 Sclera

The sclera is the protective, fibrous, white coat of the eye composed of type I collagen. It is formed from the mesenchyme during embryonic development. It extends from the corneoscleral limbus anteriorly (*Figure 2.13*) to the optic nerve posteriorly (where it is at its thickest at 1.0mm). It is covered by the conjunctiva and Tenon's capsule, and serves as the insertion for the EOM (where it is at its thinnest at 0.3mm). Between Tenon's capsule and the sclera, there is the episclera, which is a layer of loose, vascular, fibroelastic tissue. Like the cornea, the sclera is avascular, but its nutritional supply is from the episcleral layers superiorly (supplied by the anterior ciliary arteries, and the long and short posterior ciliary arteries), and the choroid that lies inferiorly.

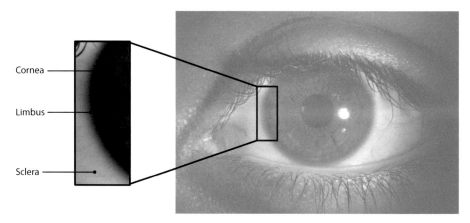

Cornea

Limbus

Sclera

Figure 2.13 Corneoscleral limbus – the junction between the cornea and sclera.

CLINICAL CONTEXT TIPS

How to examine the conjunctiva and sclera
- Ask the patient to look up, down, left and right, whilst holding the eyelids (*Figure 2.14*).
- Use a pen torch for better visualization.
- Use fluorescein 2% and a blue cobalt light to assess continuity.
- Observe for:
  - redness
  - foreign body
  - areas of scleral rupture in trauma (do you see a break in the sclera or dark uveal tissue prolapse through a break?) can occur at the corneoscleral limbus and posterior to the EOM insertion
- Note, posterior sclera cannot be assessed with this technique.

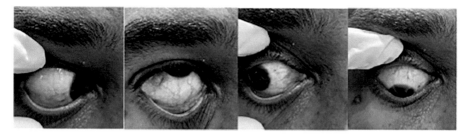

Figure 2.14 Visualization of the four quadrants of the sclera and conjunctiva (left to right: temporal, inferior, nasal, superior).

2.7 Anterior chamber and iridocorneal angle

The anterior chamber (*Figure 2.15*) is a space between the endothelium of the cornea and the iris. Its depth varies from person to person, but the average anterior chamber depth (ACD) is approximately 3–4mm, and it has a volume of approximately 250µl. Hyperopic (far-sighted) patients often have a reduced ACD compared with myopic (near-sighted) patients.

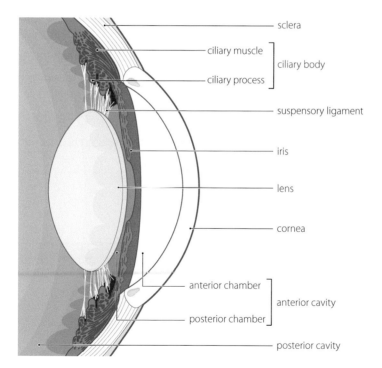

Figure 2.15 Cross-section through the eye showing the anterior and posterior chambers. Reproduced from Marshall, P. *et al.* (2017) *Anatomy and Physiology in Healthcare*. Scion Publishing Ltd.

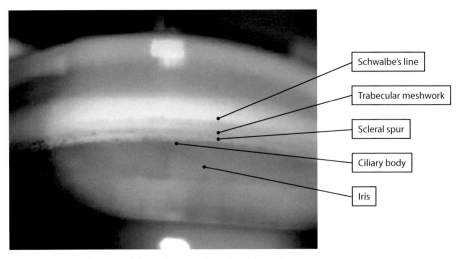

Figure 2.16 Visualization of the iridocorneal angle with gonioscopy.

The anterior chamber is filled with aqueous humour, which maintains the anterior chamber space and the intraocular pressure. The aqueous humour also provides nutrition and immunoglobulins for any immune response required for the avascular cornea. The aqueous humour is produced by the ciliary body at a rate of 2–2.5µl per minute.

The iridocorneal angle is a complex of structures which function to maintain the intraocular pressure of the globe. These structures are only visible during gonioscopy, which uses a special lens on the slit lamp to visualize the structures of the iridocorneal angle (*Figure 2.16*). In an anterior to posterior direction, the iridocorneal angle comprises the following structures:
- Schwalbe's line – this represents the termination of Descemet's layer of the cornea
- Trabecular meshwork – this is responsible for drainage of aqueous fluid from the anterior chamber
- Scleral spur
- Ciliary body – this consists of the ciliary muscle and epithelium
- Iris.

This angle is bordered anteriorly by the cornea and sclera, and posteriorly by the iris root and the anterior surface of the ciliary body.

The ciliary body has three main functions:
- Accommodation – adjusting the eye to allow it to focus on near objects
- Production and resorption of aqueous humour
- Providing an anchor for the zonules of the lens (see *Section 2.8*).

Embryonically, the ciliary body originates from the neuroepithelium. Nerve innervation is via the parasympathetic (CN III via the ciliary ganglion) and sympathetic nervous systems, and both of these facilitate the changing of eye focus. Vascular supply for the ciliary body consists of the anterior and long posterior ciliary arteries, which arise from the ophthalmic artery. Venous drainage is via the vortex veins, which drain into the superior and inferior orbital veins. The ciliary body comprises one-third of the uveal tract (which includes the iris and the choroid), and its inflammation and spasm results in the sensation of photophobia in uveitis (inflammation of any of the uveal tract structures).

As can be seen in *Figure 2.17*, once aqueous humour is produced by the ciliary epithelial cells ①, it passes through the posterior chamber via the pupil ②, drains through the trabecular meshwork into Schlemm's canal ③, and then via collector channels to the episcleral veins. A minor pathway, the uveoscleral pathway, also contributes to aqueous outflow, where aqueous humour passes through to the supraciliary and suprachoroidal space.

CLINICAL CONTEXT TIPS

How to assess the anterior chamber
Observe for:
- Depth:
  - position patient in dimly lit room
  - ask patient to fixate on a distant target
  - position pen torch laterally at the level of the iris
    - full illumination of the iris suggests a deep anterior chamber
    - crescent shadow on the nasal aspect of the iris suggests a shallow anterior chamber (*Figure 2.18*)
- Hypopyon: collection of yellow–white pus with a fluid level (see *Figures 10.1C* and *10.1D*)
- Hyphaema: collection of blood (see *Figure 16.9*).

2.8 Iris and pupil

The iris is the most anterior portion of the uveal tract. Its embryonic origin is the neuroepithelium. Its peripheral extent is attached to the ciliary body, whilst it extends centrally to form a border that makes up the pupil. The iris separates the anterior and posterior chambers (see *Figure 2.15*). The iris is divided into a central pupillary zone and a peripheral ciliary zone by the collarettes (the thickest part of the iris) (*Figure 2.19*). Another feature of the iris is contraction furrows, which are circumferential folds found in the periphery of the iris which are produced as a result of contraction and dilation of the pupil. The iris comprises anterior and posterior layers, with the vessels, nerves and sphincter pupillae being found in the anterior layer, and the dilator pupillae found in the posterior layer. The vascular supply to the iris is mainly derived from the anterior ciliary and long posterior ciliary arteries, whilst venous drainage is via the vortex veins. A non-circular iris may be due to trauma or surgery. Dilated blood vessels on the surface of the iris can be an indication of ocular inflammation. New blood vessels on the iris can be a sign of ischaemic retinopathy (caused, for example, by poorly controlled diabetes).

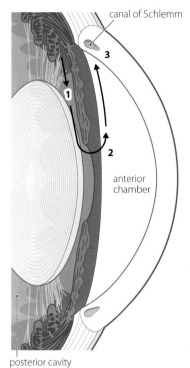

canal of Schlemm

3

1

2

anterior
chamber

posterior cavity

Figure 2.17 Conventional outflow pathway for aqueous humour via the trabecular meshwork.
① Production of the aqueous humour by the ciliary body. ② Passage of the aqueous humour through the pupil. ③ Aqueous humour drains from the trabecular meshwork into Schlemm's canal. Reproduced from Marshall, P. *et al.* (2017) *Anatomy and Physiology in Healthcare*. Scion Publishing Ltd.

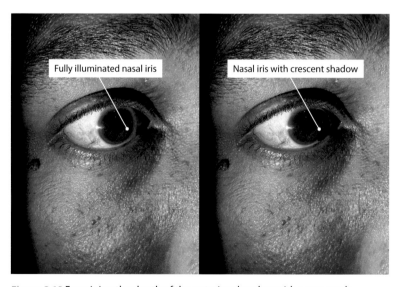

Fully illuminated nasal iris

Nasal iris with crescent shadow

Figure 2.18 Examining the depth of the anterior chamber with a pen torch.

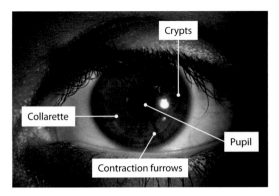

Figure 2.19 Iris and pupil.

The sphincter and dilator pupillae iris muscles control the size of the pupil, to either limit or enhance the amount of light entering the eye, respectively. The parasympathetic nervous system controls the sphincter muscle, whilst the sympathetic nervous system controls the dilator muscle.

CLINICAL CONTEXT TIPS

How to assess the pupils
Observe for:
- Colour
- Size
- Shape
- Position
- Asymmetry in size between pupils, in dim and bright light (anisocoria)
- Direct and consensual responses
- Relative afferent pupillary defect.

Figure 2.20 demonstrates how to assess for pupillary reflexes.

Step 1: Assess the pupil in dim and bright lighting, looking for **S**ize, **S**hape, **P**osition, **A**symmetry (one pupil looks different to the other). Note: in patients with dark irises, you are likely to need a dim secondary light to visualize the pupils (*Figure 2.20A*).

Step 2: Assess for direct and consensual pupil responses. The direct response (*Figure 2.20B*) is tested by shining light directly at the eye and expecting the pupil to constrict. The consensual response (*Figure 2.20C*) is tested by shining light directly at the eye and observing the contralateral eye constricting.

Step 3: Test for relative afferent pupillary defect (RAPD) (*Figure 2.20D*). The affected pupil dilates when you move the light from one eye to the other. Shine light in one

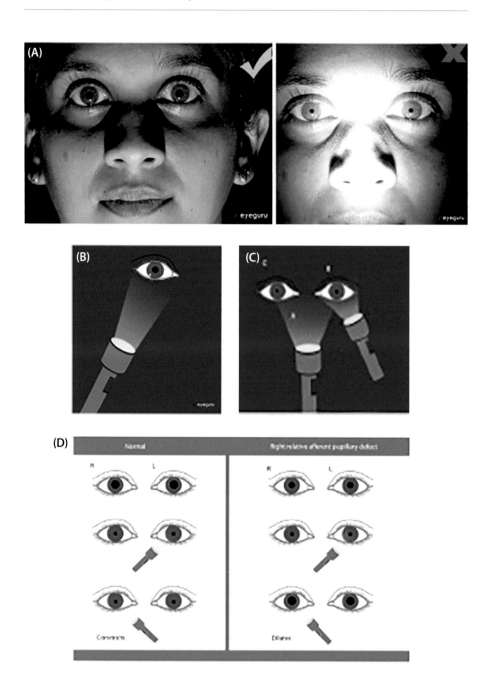

Figure 2.20 Examination of the pupils. (A) Assessing the pupils in dim and bright light. (B) Testing for direct pupil response. (C) Testing for consensual pupil response. (D) Testing for relative afferent pupillary defect. Images reproduced from https://eyeguru.org/blog/examining-the-pupil/, with permission.

eye for 3 seconds, then shine the light in the other eye for 3 seconds, then shine in the 'starting eye' again and observe its reaction. If it dilates, there is an RAPD present in that eye.

2.9 Lens

The lens is a biconvex structure (*Figure 2.21*) which contributes approximately one-third of the refractive (focusing) power of the eye. It is formed from the surface ectoderm and consists of a cortex and nucleus, enveloped by a lens epithelium which is covered by an acellular capsule. The anterior capsule is thicker than the posterior capsule, and the transparency of the lens is maintained by the lack of blood vessels and cellular structures, as well as tightly packed proteins that make up the lens fibres.

The suspensory ligaments (also known as zonules) of the lens are attached to the ciliary body (see *Figure 2.15*), and these allow the lens shape to change in order to change the eye focus. The anteroposterior diameter of the lens is approximately 4.3mm, but this increases with accommodation. The posterior surface is more convex than the anterior surface.

CLINICAL CONTEXT TIPS

How to assess the lens
The clarity of the lens can be assessed with the direct ophthalmoscope by analysing the symmetry of the red reflex (the reflection of light from the retina, as viewed through a direct ophthalmoscope or retinoscope; see *Figure 15.3*).

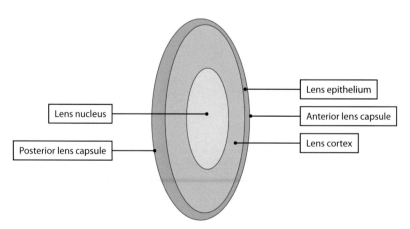

Figure 2.21 Schematic diagram of the lens.

2.10 Posterior segment

The posterior segment spans from the posterior aspect of the crystalline lens and incorporates the vitreous humour (the gel that fills the back of the eye), retina (the film that collects the 'visual information' from the environment), choroid (the nutritious vascular layer) and optic nerve (the nerve which connects the eye to the brain).

The posterior pole consists of the optic disc ('head' of the optic nerve), macula (centre of the retina) and fovea (centre of the macula responsible for the best central fine vision) which is bordered by superior and inferior temporal vascular arcades (*Figure 2.22*). During fundoscopy, a healthy fovea will exhibit a foveal reflex, where light from the ophthalmoscope or slit lamp is reflected from the fovea and the observer views a pinpoint of light over the fovea.

The vitreous humour is mainly water (99%) and collagen, and fills the space between the posterior aspect of the lens and the retina. Embryonically, it originates from the extracellular mesenchyme. It has an average volume of 4ml. Its function is to maintain the shape of the eye, as well as providing a transparent medium that allows passage of light to the retina. It is firmly attached at the vitreous base, an area overlying the ora serrata, and at the optic disc. The ora serrata is the transition point between the retina and the ciliary body epithelium, and where the retina is firmly attached in the periphery.

The retina and the optic nerves originate from the neuroepithelium, whilst the choroid originates from the mesenchyme (like the sclera). The retina is divided into the neurosensory retina and the retinal pigment epithelium, and both layers are continuous with the ciliary body epithelium at the ora serrata. The neurosensory retina

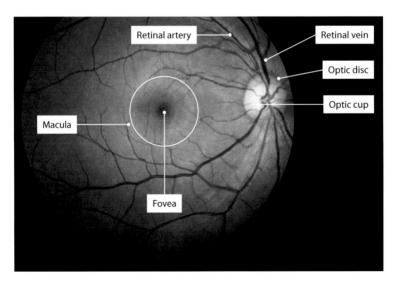

Figure 2.22 Structures of the posterior pole.

contains the apparatus necessary to convert visual information from the environment to impulses that are transported via the optic disc to the brain so that they can be interpreted. Its embryonic origin is the inner layer of the neuroectoderm, and it has an average diameter of 200µm, although it is thinner at the periphery. The apparatus required for retinal function includes photoreceptors, bipolar cells and ganglion cells, and modulating cells such as horizontal cells (*Figure 2.23*).

There are two types of photoreceptors in the retina, rods and cones, and there are twice as many rods as there are cones. The highest concentration of cones is at the fovea and these cones are necessary for central and colour vision (fine detail). The rods are important for peripheral vision and vision in low light. The retinal pigment epithelium (RPE) is a layer of epithelial cells that is instrumental in maintaining the physiological function of the neurosensory retina. Posterior to the RPE is Bruch's membrane and the choroid, the latter being a highly vascular structure. There is a dual blood supply to the retina, with the inner retina (up to the inner nuclear layer) supplied by the central retinal artery (which is a branch of the ophthalmic artery), and the outer retina (from the inner nuclear layer to the RPE / Bruch membrane complex) supplied by the choroidal circulation (subsidiaries of the short posterior ciliary arteries).

CLINICAL CONTEXT TIPS

How to assess the posterior segment
Visualization of the posterior segment outside of the ophthalmology clinic is difficult without experience. The best visualization usually requires pupil dilation, but it is still possible to visualize the posterior pole including the optic disc, the superior and inferior vascular arcades and the fovea with the direct ophthalmoscope and an undilated pupil in a dimly lit room. Furthermore, symmetry of the red reflex can also give clues to posterior segment pathology.

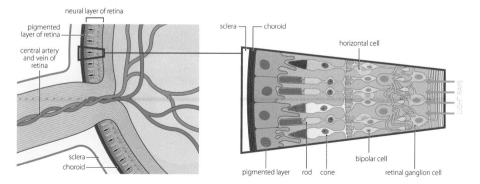

Figure 2.23 Cross-sectional diagram of the retina. Reproduced from Marshall, P. *et al.* (2017) *Anatomy and Physiology in Healthcare*. Scion Publishing Ltd.

Chapter 3
Common terminology and abbreviations used in an ophthalmological report

3.1 Introduction

There are a number of terms found on most ophthalmology reports that appear as a result of preset functions in electronic patient records (EPR). The following is a list of abbreviations, key words and phrases which appear frequently in ophthalmology reports. Knowing these will help with decoding and understanding letters and reports from the eye clinic.

For general abbreviations, see the list that appears just before *Chapter 1*.

3.2 Common terms

AAC/ACG/AACG	acute angle closure / angle closure glaucoma / acute angle closure glaucoma
AC	anterior chamber
ACIOL	anterior chamber intraocular lens
ACT	alternate cover test
AAION	arteritic anterior ischaemic optic neuropathy
AION	anterior ischaemic optic neuropathy
AMD	age-related macular degeneration
anti-VEGF	anti-vascular endothelial growth factor
APD	afferent pupillary defect
BCL	bandage contact lens
BCVA	best corrected visual acuity
BRAO	branch retinal artery occlusion
BRVO	branch retinal vein occlusion
cc	with refractive correction (i.e. with glasses / contact lenses on)
CCT	central corneal thickness
C/D	cup–disc ratio
CMO	cystoid macular oedema
CNV	choroidal neovascularization

CNVM	choroidal neovascular membrane
COAG	chronic open angle glaucoma
CRAO	central retinal artery occlusion
CRVO	central retinal vein occlusion
CRx	cycloplegic refraction
CSMO	clinically significant macular oedema
CSR	central serous retinopathy
CT	cover test
CV	colour vision
CWS	cotton wool spot
Cyl	cylinder (measure of astigmatism)
DALK	deep anterior lamellar keratoplasty, aka corneal anterior lamellar graft (a form of corneal transplant that helps improve corneal clarity and vision)
DFE	dilated fundus examination
DMO	diabetic macular oedema
DSEK/DMEK	Descemet's stripping (automated) endothelial keratoplasty / Descemet's membrane endothelial keratoplasty, aka corneal endothelial graft (a form of corneal transplant that helps improve corneal clarity and vision)
E	esophoria (a type of strabismus / eye misalignment with inward eye deviation which is only present when the eye is covered)
ECCE	extracapsular cataract extraction
EOG	electrooculogram
EOM	extraocular muscle
Epiphora	watery eye
ERG	electroretinogram
ERM	epiretinal membrane
ET	esotropia (a type of strabismus / eye misalignment with inward eye deviation which is always present)
E(T)	intermittent esotropia
FB	foreign body
FDT	forced duction test (assesses eye muscle function)
FDDT	fluorescein dye disappearance test (assesses patency of the tear duct system)
F&F	fix and follow
FFA	fundus fluorescein angiography (a form of 'X-ray' test to allow visualization of the retinal blood vessels – see Chapter 20)

FTMH	full thickness macular hole
g	gutta (drops)
GAT	Goldmann applanation tonometer (measures intraocular pressure)
GCA	giant cell arteritis
GVF	Goldmann visual field
HT	hypertropia (a type of strabismus / eye misalignment with upward eye deviation which is always present)
H(T)	intermittent hypertropia
HVF	Humphrey visual field
HypoT	hypotropia (a type of strabismus / eye misalignment with downward eye deviation which is always present)
Hypo(T)	intermittent hypotropia
iCare	contact method of measuring intraocular pressure
IOFB	intraocular foreign body
ION	ischaemic optic neuropathy
IOP	intraocular pressure
IPD	interpupillary distance
Ishihara test	method of assessing colour vision
KCN	keratoconus
KP	keratic precipitates
LASIK	laser *in situ* keratomileusis (laser refractive surgery)
LogMAR	log of minimum angle of resolution (unit measure for visual acuity)
LOV	loss of vision
LPI	laser peripheral iridotomy (laser treatment for pupillary block in AAC or to prevent pupillary block in narrow angle glaucoma)
MIGS	microinvasive glaucoma surgery
NAION	non-arteritic anterior ischaemic optic neuropathy
NIPH	no improvement with pinhole (when measuring visual acuity)
NPDR	non-proliferative diabetic retinopathy
NPL	no perception of light
NSC	nuclear sclerosis cataract
NTG	normal tension glaucoma
NVA	neovascularization of the angle
NVD	neovascularization at the disc
NVE	neovascularization elsewhere
NVG	neovascular glaucoma
NVI	neovascularization of the iris

oc	oculentum (ointment)
OCT	optical coherence tomography
OHT	ocular hypertension
PCIOL	posterior chamber intraocular lens
PCO	posterior capsular opacification
PDR	proliferative diabetic retinopathy
PEE	punctate epithelial erosion
ph	pinhole (when measuring visual acuity)
Phaco + IOL	cataract extraction via phacoemulsification plus intraocular lens implantation
PK	penetrating keratoplasty (full thickness corneal transplant)
POAG	primary open angle glaucoma
PRP	panretinal photocoagulation
PSC	posterior subcapsular cataract
PVD	posterior vitreous detachment
RAPD	relative afferent pupillary defect
RD	retinal detachment
ROP	retinopathy of prematurity
sc	without correction with glasses or contact lens
SCH	subconjunctival haemorrhage
SLT	selective laser trabeculoplasty (laser treatment for open angle glaucoma)
Snellen chart	chart used to assess visual acuity
TBUT	tear break-up time (for assessing tear film quality)
Tonopen	contact method of measuring intraocular pressure
VA	visual acuity
VF	visual field
VH	vitreous haemorrhage
VMT	vitreomacular traction
X	exophoria (a type of strabismus / eye misalignment with outward eye deviation which is only present when the eye is covered)
XT	exotropia (a type of strabismus / eye misalignment with outward eye deviation which is always present)
X(T)	intermittent exotropia
YAG Caps	YAG laser capsulotomy – laser treatment for posterior capsular opacification of an intraocular lens

Chapter 4
Common ophthalmic medications

4.1 Introduction

The eye clinic utilizes a number of diagnostic and therapeutic drops. As always, the *British National Formulary* (*BNF*) is the essential reference for the required dosage of the drops and other medications used in ophthalmology. However, the following is a quick reference list of key and common ophthalmic medications and their indications.

> Please consult your local hospital policies and formulary for the availability and recommended doses of these medications.

4.2 Key medications and their indications

Acetazolamide

Indication: Raised intraocular pressure
Mode of action: Suppresses aqueous humour production
Preparation: Tablet (*slow release (SR) or prolonged release (PR)*) or IV
Trade name(s): Diamox

Acetylcysteine 5%

Indication: Filamentary keratitis; severe dry eye
Mode of action: Mucolytic
Preparation: Eye drop
Trade name(s): Ilube (combined with hypromellose)

Aciclovir 3%

Indication: Viral keratitis
Mode of action: Viral DNA polymerase inhibitor and disrupts viral DNA synthesis
Preparation: Eye ointment
Trade name(s): Aciclovir Agepha 30mg/g

Amphotericin

Indication: Fungal keratitis (yeast-like fungi)
Mode of action: Increases fungal cell wall permeability
Preparation: Eye drop (0.15%), intracameral (5–10 micrograms in 0.1ml) or intravitreal (10 micrograms in 0.1ml) injection
Trade name(s): n/a

Anti-VEGF (vascular endothelial retinal growth factor)

Indication:	Age-related macular degeneration; macular oedema (diabetic retinopathy, vein occlusions, cystoid macular oedema); proliferative retinopathy; retinopathy of prematurity; choroidal neovascularization
Mode of action:	Inhibits binding of VEGF to its receptors
Preparation:	Intravitreal injection
Trade name(s):	Eylea (aflibercept), Lucentis (ranibizumab), Avastin (bevacizumab, off-label use), Beovu (brolucizumab)

Apraclonidine 0.5% / 1%

Indication:	Raised intraocular pressure / glaucoma management
Mode of action:	Alpha-2 adrenergic receptor agonist which reduces aqueous humour production and increases aqueous humour outflow via the uveoscleral pathway
Preparation:	Eye drop
Trade name(s):	Iopidine

Atropine 1%

Indication:	Pupil dilation
Mode of action:	Muscarinic antagonist
Preparation:	Eye drop
Trade name(s):	n/a

Azelastine 0.05%

Indication:	Anti-allergy
Mode of action:	Selective histamine H_1 antagonist (second generation)
Preparation:	Eye drop
Trade name(s):	Optilast

Azithromycin

Indication:	Bacterial and chlamydial conjunctivitis
Mode of action:	Macrolide that inhibits bacterial protein synthesis (bacteriostatic)
Preparation:	Eye drop (1.5%)
Trade name(s):	Azyter 15mg/g

Betamethasone 0.1%

Indication:	Anti-inflammatory
Mode of action:	Controls synthesis of inflammatory mediators
Preparation:	Eye drop and ointment
Trade name(s):	n/a

Betaxolol 0.25% / 0.5%

Indication:	Raised intraocular pressure / glaucoma management
Mode of action:	Beta-blocker suppressing aqueous humour production
Preparation:	Eye drop
Trade name(s):	Betoptic

Bimatoprost 0.01% / 0.03%
Indication: Raised intraocular pressure / glaucoma management
Mode of action: Increases aqueous humour outflow
Preparation: Eye drop
Trade name(s):   Lumigan

Brimonidine 0.2%
Indication: Raised intraocular pressure / glaucoma management
Mode of action: Alpha-2 adrenergic receptor agonist which reduces aqueous humour production and increases aqueous humour outflow via the uveoscleral pathway
Preparation: Eye drop
Trade name(s):   Alphagan

Brinzolamide 1%
Indication: Raised intraocular pressure / glaucoma management
Mode of action: Suppresses aqueous humour production
Preparation: Eye drop
Trade name(s):   Azopt

Bromfenac 0.09%
Indication: Post-operative inflammation after cataract surgery
Mode of action: Inhibition of cyclooxygenase (mainly COX-2) and prostaglandin synthesis
Preparation: Eye drop
Trade name(s):   Yellox

Carteolol
Indication: Raised intraocular pressure / glaucoma management
Mode of action: Beta-blocker suppressing aqueous humour production
Preparation: Eye drop
Trade name(s):   Teoptic

Cefuroxime
Indication: Bacterial keratitis
Mode of action: Disruption of production of bacterial cell wall (bactericidal)
Preparation: Eye drop (5%), intracameral (1mg/0.1ml)
Trade name(s):   n/a

Chloramphenicol
Indication: Bacterial eye infection
Mode of action: Inhibits bacterial protein synthesis (bactericidal and bacteriostatic)
Preparation: Eye drop (0.5%) or ointment (1%)
Trade name(s):   n/a

Chlorhexidine 0.02%
Indication: *Acanthamoeba* keratitis
Mode of action: Biguanide that inhibits membrane function (bactericidal)
Preparation: Eye drop
Trade name(s):   n/a

Ciclosporin 0.1%

Indication:	Severe dry eye; vernal keratoconjunctivitis
Mode of action:	Immunosuppressant
Preparation:	Eye drop
Trade name(s):	Ikervis, Verkazia

Ciprofloxacin 0.3%

Indication:	Corneal ulcer and bacterial conjunctivitis
Mode of action:	Fluoroquinolone that inhibits DNA gyrase and therefore bacterial DNA synthesis (bactericidal)
Preparation:	Eye drop
Trade name(s):	Ciloxan

Cyclopentolate 0.5% / 1%

Indication:	Pupil dilation
Mode of action:	Muscarinic antagonist
Preparation:	Eye drop: 0.5% for children under the age of 1 year; 1% for patients aged 1 year and above
Trade name(s):	Mydrilate

Dexamethasone

Indication:	Uveitis; post-operative anti-inflammatory
Mode of action:	Controls synthesis of inflammatory mediators
Preparation:	Eye drop
Trade name(s):	Maxidex (0.1%), Dropdex, Dexafree, Ozurdex (intravitreal implant 700 micrograms)

Diclofenac sodium 0.1%

Indication:	Post-operative anti-inflammatory
Mode of action:	Inhibits prostaglandin synthesis
Preparation:	Eye drop
Trade name(s):	Voltarol Ophtha

Dorzolamide 2%

Indication:	Raised intraocular pressure / glaucoma management
Mode of action:	Suppresses aqueous humour production
Preparation:	Eye drop
Trade name(s):	Trusopt, Vizidor, Eylamdo

Econazole 1%

Indication:	Fungal keratitis
Mode of action:	Disruption of fungal cell wall synthesis
Preparation:	Eye drop
Trade name(s):	n/a

Erythromycin (0.5%)

Indication:	Bacterial conjunctivitis, ophthalmia neonatorum
Mode of action:	Macrolide that inhibits bacterial protein synthesis (bacteriostatic)
Preparation:	Topical drops, ointment or tablet
Trade name(s):	n/a

Fluocinolone acetonide

Indication: Diabetic macula oedema, non-infectious uveitis
Mode of action: Controls synthesis of inflammatory mediators
Preparation: Intravitreal implant
Trade name(s):   Iluvien

Fluoromethalone 0.1%

Indication: Anti-inflammatory
Mode of action: Controls synthesis of inflammatory mediators
Preparation: Eye drop
Trade name(s):   FML

Fusidic acid 1%

Indication: Bacterial conjunctivitis
Mode of action: Inhibits bacterial DNA translation (bacteriostatic)
Preparation: Eye gel
Trade name(s):   Fucidin

Ganciclovir 0.15%

Indication: Viral keratitis
Mode of action: Inhibits viral replication
Preparation: Eye gel
Trade name(s):   Virgan

Gentamicin 0.3%

Indication: Bacterial keratitis and corneal ulcer
Mode of action: Aminoglycoside that inhibits protein synthesis (bactericidal)
Preparation: Eye drop
Trade name(s):   n/a

Hydrocortisone

Indication: Anti-inflammatory
Mode of action: Controls synthesis of inflammatory mediators
Preparation: Preservative-free eye drop
Trade name(s):   Softacort

Ketorolac 0.5%

Indication: Post-operative anti-inflammatory
Mode of action: Inhibits cyclooxygenase
Preparation: Eye drop
Trade name(s):   Acular

Ketotifen

Indication: Allergic conjunctivitis
Mode of action: Non-competitive H_1 antihistamine and mast cell stabilizer
Preparation: Eye drop
Trade name(s):   Zaditor

Latanoprost 0.05%

Indication:	Raised intraocular pressure / glaucoma management
Mode of action:	Increases aqueous humour outflow
Preparation:	Eye drop
Trade name(s):	Xalatan, Monoprost

Levobunolol

Indication:	Raised intraocular pressure / glaucoma management
Mode of action:	Beta-blocker suppressing aqueous humour production
Preparation:	Eye drop
Trade name(s):	Betagan

Levofloxacin 0.5%

Indication:	Bacterial keratitis; contact lens related keratitis
Mode of action:	Fluoroquinolone that inhibits DNA gyrase and therefore bacterial DNA synthesis (bactericidal)
Preparation:	Eye drop
Trade name(s):	Oftaquix, Oxalux

Lodoxamide

Indication:	Anti-allergy
Mode of action:	Mast cell stabilizer
Preparation:	Eye drop
Trade name(s):	Alomide

Loteprednol 0.5%

Indication:	Anti-inflammatory
Mode of action:	Controls synthesis of inflammatory mediators
Preparation:	Eye drop
Trade name(s):	Lotemax

Mannitol

Indication:	Recalcitrant raised intraocular pressure in acute glaucoma; pre-operative in complicated cataract operations
Mode of action:	Dehydrates the vitreous humour
Preparation:	Intravenous infusion
Trade name(s):	n/a

Miconazole 1%

Indication:	Fungal keratitis
Mode of action:	Disruption of fungal cell wall synthesis
Preparation:	Eye drop
Trade name(s):	n/a

Miochol

Indication:	Rapid intraoperative miosis
Mode of action:	Cholinergic agonist
Preparation:	Instillation solution, acetylcholine chloride
Trade name(s):	Miochol-E

Moxifloxacin 0.5%
Indication: Bacterial keratitis; contact lens related keratitis
Mode of action: Fluoroquinolone that inhibits DNA gyrase and therefore bacterial
                   DNA synthesis (bactericidal)
Preparation: Eye drop
Trade name(s):   Moxivig

Natamycin 1%
Indication: Fungal (filamentous fungi) keratitis
Mode of action: Disruption of fungal cell walls
Preparation: Eye drop
Trade name(s):   Natacyn

Nepafenac 0.1% / 0.3%
Indication: Cystoid macular oedema in diabetic patients after cataract surgery;
                   post-operative inflammation
Mode of action: Non-steroidal anti-inflammatory
Preparation: Eye drop
Trade name(s):   Nevanac

Ofloxacin 0.3%
Indication: Bacterial keratitis; contact lens related keratitis
Mode of action: A fluoroquinolone that inhibits DNA gyrase and therefore bacterial
                   DNA synthesis (bactericidal)
Preparation: Eye drop
Trade name(s):   Exocin

Olopatadine 0.1%
Indication: Anti-allergy
Mode of action: Histamine H_1 antagonist (second generation)
Preparation: Eye drop
Trade name(s):   Pataday, Opatanol

Oxybuprocaine 0.4%
Indication: Topical anaesthetic
Mode of action: Decreases the permeability of the neuronal membrane to sodium
                   ions
Preparation: Eye drop
Trade name(s):   n/a

Phenylephrine 2.5% / 10%
Indication: Pupil dilation; blanch test for episcleritis / scleritis
Mode of action: Alpha adrenergic agonist
Preparation: Eye drop
Trade name(s):   n/a

Pilocarpine 1% / 2% / 4%
Indication: To stop pupillary block in acute angle closure glaucoma; chronic
                     glaucoma; miosis; diagnosis of Horner's syndrome (diluted)
Mode of action: Direct-acting cholinergic agonist
Preparation: Eye drop
Trade name(s):   n/a

Polyhexamethylene
Indication: *Acanthamoeba* corneal infections
Mode of action: Biguanide that inhibits membrane function (bactericidal)
Preparation: 0.02% and 0.06% eye drop
Trade name(s):   PHMB

Prednisolone 0.5% / 1%
Indication: Anti-inflammatory
Mode of action: Controls synthesis of inflammatory mediators
Preparation: Eye drop
Trade name(s):   Pred Forte 1%, Minims Prednisolone Sodium Phosphate 0.5%

Propamidine isetionate
Indication: *Acanthamoeba* corneal infections
Mode of action: Diamidine that inhibits DNA synthesis (bacteriostatic)
Preparation: 0.1% eye drop
Trade name(s):   Brolene

Proxymetacaine 0.5%
Indication: Topical anaesthetic
Mode of action: Decreases the permeability of the neuronal membrane to sodium ions
Preparation: Eye drop
Trade name(s):   n/a

Sodium cromoglicate
Indication: Allergic conjunctivitis
Mode of action: Mast cell stabilizer
Preparation: Eye drop
Trade name(s):   Allercrom, Catacrom, Opticrom, Eycrom

Tafluprost
Indication: Glaucoma
Mode of action: Increase aqueous humour outflow
Preparation: Preservative-free eye drop
Trade name(s):   Saflutan

Tetracaine 0.5%
Indication: Topical anaesthetic
Mode of action: Decreases the permeability of the neuronal membrane to sodium ions
Preparation: Eye drop
Trade name(s):   n/a

Timolol 0.1% / 0.25% / 0.5%

Indication:	Raised intraocular pressure / glaucoma management
Mode of action:	Beta-blocker suppressing aqueous humour production
Preparation:	Eye drop or gel
Trade name(s):	Tiopex (0.1%), Timoptol LA (long-acting), Eysano (0.25% or 0.5%) preservative-free

Travoprost 0.004%

Indication:	Raised intraocular pressure / glaucoma management
Mode of action:	Increases aqueous humour outflow at the trabecular meshwork
Preparation:	Eye drop
Trade name(s):	Travatan

Triamcinolone

Indication:	Anti-inflammatory
Mode of action:	Controls synthesis of inflammatory mediators
Preparation:	Intravitreal, intracameral
Trade name(s):	Intracinol

Tropicamide 0.5% / 1%

Indication:	Pupil dilation
Mode of action	Anticholinergic
Preparation:	Eye drop
Trade name(s):	Mydriacyl

Voriconazole 1%

Indication:	Fungal keratitis
Mode of action:	Disruption of fungal cell wall synthesis
Preparation:	Eye drop
Trade name(s):	n/a

4.3 Combination glaucoma drops

Trade name	Components
Azarga	Brinzolamide with timolol
Combigan	Brimonidine with timolol
Cosopt, Eylamdo, Tidomat	Dorzolamide with timolol
DuoTrav	Travoprost with timolol
Fixapost, Xalacom	Latanoprost with timolol
Ganfort	Bimatoprost with timolol
Simbrinza	Brinzolamide with brimonidine
Taptiqom	Tafluprost with timolol

4.4 Dry eyes drops / lubricating eye drops

Drops	Trade name(s)
Carbomer (0.2%)	Clinitas
Carmellose sodium (0.5% / 1%)	Carmize, Cellusan, Celluvisc, Evolve, Xailin Fresh
Hypromellose (0.3%)	Artelac, Brolene Cool, Hydromoor, Hypromol, Isopto Plain, Lumecare, Xailin Hydrate
Paraffin-based	Lacri-Lube, Hylo Night, Xailin Night
Polyvinyl alcohol (1.4%)	Liquifilm Tears, Sno Tears
Propylene glycol 0.3% and polyethylene glycol 0.4%	Systane preservative-free, Systane Balance
Sodium hyaluronate (0.1% / 0.2% / 0.4%)	Aeon Protect, Artelac Splash, Artelac Rebalance, Blink Intensive, Eyezin XL, Hyabak, Hycosan, HydraMed, Hylo-Care, Hylo-Forte, Hylo-Tear, Hy-Opti, Lubristil, Ocu-Lube HA, Ocusan, Oftaox, Optive Fusion, Thealoz Duo, Vismed, Xailin HA

4.5 Other combination ocular medications

Trade name(s)	Components
Betnesol N	Betamethasone and neomycin
Maxitrol	Dexamethasone, neomycin, polymyxin
Mydrane	Tropicamide, lidocaine, phenylephrine
Mydriasert	Phenylephrine and tropicamide
Sofradex	Dexamethasone, framycetin, gramicidin

Chapter 5
Focusing your history: sorting the symptoms

5.1 Introduction

How to take a basic ophthalmology history was covered in *Chapter 1*. This chapter will cover further relevant symptoms which may lead you to one diagnosis over another for acute ophthalmic presenting complaints (signs and symptoms occurring for 0–4 days). The suggested diagnoses are what is *most likely*, given the symptoms described by the patient.

5.2 Red eye

Red eye is usually a front of the eye problem and it can present in a variety of ways.

5.2.1 Bloodshot but painless eye

Usually incidentally noticed by a relative or patient looking in the mirror – a (usually) unilateral bright red eye ➞ subconjunctival haemorrhage.

5.2.2 Bloodshot but painful eye

The patient had recent trauma or eyelid or orbital surgery; taking blood thinners: unilateral diffusely red eye, with proptosis ➞ retrobulbar haemorrhage

5.2.3 Both eyes affected with irritation / soreness

- Dry / gritty eyes, water in the wind ➞ dry eye
- With crusting in morning (vision feels like it has an oily film over it, and more chronic) ➞ blepharitis
- With bilateral lid swelling ➞ conjunctivitis (or blepharoconjunctivitis if associated with blepharitis)
  - with watery discharge ➞ allergy (especially if itchy) or viral infection (especially if recent upper respiratory tract infection)
  - with purulent discharge (and usually more unilateral) ➞ bacterial infection

5.2.4 Irritation

Typically unilateral (but may occur in both eyes) with sectoral redness ➞ episcleritis

5.2.5 Deep ache

Unilateral with deep redness, which wakes the patient at night ➞ scleritis (especially if known underlying autoimmune condition).

How to differentiate scleritis from episcleritis
- Episcleritis:
  - sectoral redness (though occasionally can be diffuse)
  - less symptomatic (more uncomfortable than painful)
  - superficial vessels involved, easily move with cotton bud
  - redness blanches on 2.5% phenylephrine instillation
  - non-tender globe
  - is not usually associated with systemic disease.

5.2.6 Foreign body sensation or severe searing pain

This is most likely related to corneal pathology:
- Recent trauma → corneal abrasion, foreign body, microbial keratitis, chemical injury
- Worse on waking especially if previous trauma → recurrent corneal erosion syndrome
- Contact lens wearer → contact lens keratitis

5.2.7 Photosensitivity

This is most likely to be a corneal or uveal pathology (see below for how to differentiate).

How to differentiate between corneal and uveal pathology
- Corneal – look at the cornea and stain it to look for abrasions, foreign bodies and ulcers
- Uveal – look in the anterior chamber (and the fundus) for signs of intraocular inflammation.

5.2.8 Periocular rash

This is most likely to be herpetic (remember to assess for level of intraocular involvement):
- If the rash respects the midline, confined to the forehead (V1 distribution) → herpes zoster (look out for rash on the apex or lateral aspect of the nose (Hutchinson's sign) which raises suspicion of ocular involvement)
- If the rash is periorbital and typically in a patient under 50 years → herpes simplex

5.2.9 Haloes

When accompanied by vision disturbance or loss → acute angle closure

5.2.10 Post-operative / injection

When accompanied by markedly reduced vision and discharge ➞ endophthalmitis

5.3 Acute loss of vision

Acute loss of vision is usually a back of the eye problem and it is important to establish if the problem is arising at:
- the interface between the vitreous jelly and retina
- the retina
- the optic nerve.

It is also important to establish if the loss of vision is pre- or post-operative.

5.3.1 Vitreous jelly / retina interface

'Flashes and floaters' symptoms (see *Section 5.4* for more details).

5.3.2 Retina

Usually an acute loss of vision, but can also be gradual. May be vascular or macular:
- Vascular: vision loss is partial or total field loss
  - vein occlusion: older, cardiovascular risk factors
  - artery occlusion: profound acute vision loss, background of cardiovascular risk factors; beware of giant cell arteritis
- Macular: scotoma, metamorphopsia
  - if acute or gradual in an older patient ➞ age-related macular degeneration (wet)
  - diabetes causing macular pathology is less likely to be acute.

5.3.3 Optic nerve

In acute loss of vision secondary to optic neuropathies, patients often display a relative afferent pupillary defect (RAPD; *see Figure 2.20*). Generally, retinal conditions will not display an RAPD, unless more than one-third of the retina is affected, e.g. ischaemic retinal vein occlusion, central retinal artery occlusion or large retinal detachment.

Optic nerve neuropathy arises as a result of reduced blood supply or inflammation:
- Reduced blood supply ➞ ischaemic optic neuropathy
  - non-arteritic ➞ typically older patient with cardiovascular risk factors; may have an altitudinal field defect (loss of visual field in the horizontal half of visual field); test blood glucose (BG), blood pressure (BP), lipids; must rule out giant cell arteritis (see below)
  - arteritic ➞ i.e. giant cell arteritis

CLINICAL CONTEXT TIPS

How to diagnose giant cell arteritis
- Patient almost always >50 years of age
- Typical symptoms include:

- acute loss of vision (initially unilateral but beware rapid second eye involvement)
- amaurosis fugax – can be postural (ischaemia on standing)
- diplopia if cranial nerve palsies
- temporal headache
- scalp tenderness
- jaw / tongue claudication
- PMR symptoms – neck / shoulder girdle / hip pain
- systemic malaise – anorexia, weight loss, fever
- Document if any neurological / stroke symptoms
- Urgent full blood count (FBC), C-reactive protein (CRP), erythrocyte sedimentation rate (ESR)
- Consult with local giant cell arteritis protocol
- **Referrals often made to ophthalmology if presenting with ocular symptoms, and to rheumatology if presenting without ocular symptoms.**

- Inflammation
  - demyelinating, i.e. multiple-sclerosis associated, typically in young Caucasian female
  - non-infective inflammatory
  - infective, e.g. herpetic acute retinal necrosis associated
  - *compressive / infiltrative pathology is less likely to be acute.*

CLINICAL CONTEXT TIPS

Post-operative patients, particularly those who have had intraocular surgery, with acute loss of vision should be considered to have raised intraocular pressure, endophthalmitis or retinal detachment as primary differentials. These require **immediate referral** to ophthalmology.

5.4 Flashes and floaters

Patients presenting with flashes and floaters need careful assessment, but general clues to assessment are:
- 1–2 mobile floaters only ➡ vitreous syneresis
- Photopsia (flashing lights – usually in a temporal arc, more noticeable in dim light due to vitreoretinal traction) ➡ posterior vitreous detachment
- Sudden shower of floaters ➡ vitreous haemorrhage, retinal tear
- Shadow / curtain / visual field defect / loss of vision ➡ retinal detachment

5.5 Swollen lids

Swollen lids can present in one or both eyes:
- Bilateral ➡ if not blepharitis or conjunctivitis, likely to be dermatitis or angioedema

- Unilateral:
  - ○ discrete lump ➙ stye / chalazion, or benign / pre-malignant / malignant lesion
  - ○ proptosis, painful / restricted eye movements, reduced vision / colour vision, abnormal pupillary response, systemically unwell ➙ orbital cellulitis
  - ○ vesicular rash ➙ herpetic

5.6 Headaches with ringing in the ears (tinnitus) and visual obscuration

➙ raised intracranial pressure

Ask patient about:
- Character of headaches – postural or diurnal (worse on waking?)
- Nausea / vomiting
- Blurred vision
- Transient visual obscurations
- Diplopia
- Pulsatile tinnitus (whooshing / ringing / humming in the ears in sync with the heartbeat)
- Gait / speech / swallow problems.

The patient needs **immediate referral** and **admission under the medical team**. Blood tests (for pre-lumbar puncture for bleeding or clotting disorder) and urgent neuroimaging (CT/MR venograms followed by lumbar puncture if not contraindicated) should be arranged with formal dilated fundoscopy by ophthalmology to look for optic nerve swelling / papilloedema.

5.7 Transient monocular vision loss

- A 'curtain coming down' and slowly recovering within 30 minutes ➙ amaurosis fugax (a temporary loss of vision in one or both eyes due to a lack of blood flow to the retina).
  - ○ even if totally resolved: **urgent stroke team referral** for work-up and management
  - ○ any ongoing ocular symptoms: **non-urgent referral to ophthalmology**
- Are there triggers to vision loss?
  - ○ evening ➙ consider acute angle closure
  - ○ on exercise ➙ consider pigment dispersion syndrome
  - ○ on standing ➙ consider carotid insufficiency
- Rule out:
  - ○ associated neurological symptoms ➙ stroke
  - ○ crescendo amaurosis fugax, headache, temporal tenderness, jaw claudication ➙ GCA
  - ○ transient visual disturbance, GI symptoms, headache ➙ migraine-type headaches

Chapter 6

Triage ready reckoner

Whether you are referring patients to ophthalmology or triaging referrals, the guide below is designed to help you decide on the urgency with which the patient is seen by an ophthalmologist.

This is a guide only, and should not replace clinical judgement or local hospital guidance and protocols.

IR = immediate referral
SD = same day
24h = within 24 hours
48h = within 48 hours
FTC = fast-track clinic (2 week wait)
SSC = 'soon' but routine subspecialist clinic
CM = community management

SD	**3rd nerve palsy** (*new unilateral ptosis with eye depressed and abducted ± fixed dilated pupil ± pain / headache*): if diawgnosis is confirmed, refer to A&E first for same day computed tomography (CT) angiogram regardless of pain / pupil status
IR	**Acute angle closure** (*severe pain, nausea + vomiting, haloes, frontal headache, blurred vision, cloudy cornea, fixed dilated pupil*)
SD	**Acute profound vision loss**: if <6 hours or amaurosis fugax (plus stroke team referral)
CM	**Age-related macular degeneration (dry)**
FTC	**Age-related macular degeneration (wet)** (*older patient with acute distortion / acute decreased central vision*)
CM	**Blepharitis**: lid hygiene, warm compress, lubricating eye drops, consider topical antibiotic / oral antibiotic for acute flares. Refer to FTC to exclude malignancy if very unilateral or if associated corneal disease
SD	**Blunt trauma** (*hyphaema, in grafted eye, fixed dilated pupil, new floaters*)
24h	**Blunt trauma** (*with no hyphaema or new floater*)
FTC	**Cancer suspect**
SSC	**Central serous retinopathy** (*acute central distortion or scotoma usually in a young, male patient*)

CM	**Chalazion** (*sterile chronic granuloma, can flare with tender lid swelling*): treat with warm compress, use topical or oral antibiotics if pre-septal cellulitic process present; self-resolves. If recurrent or causing mechanical ptosis despite acute inflammation resolving, refer routinely to ophthalmology
IR	**Chemical injury**: start irrigation as soon as the patient presents and history elicits a chemical injury. Refer immediately to ophthalmology for assessment and management
SD	**Corneal graft patient** (*symptomatic with pain, photophobia, redness*)
CM	**Congenital nasolacrimal duct obstruction** (*infant with recurrent unilateral 'conjunctivitis', persistently watering eye, matted lashes*): instruct parents to clean the eye(s) with sterile water and cotton wool, and perform lacrimal sac massage; condition normally self-resolves by 12 months of age. Conjunctival swabs and topical antibiotics are unnecessary, unless the white of the eye itself becomes red and sore. These children are not infectious and can attend nursery. Refer routinely if concerned or not resolved by 12 months, or immediate referral in suspected ophthalmia neonatorum (infant <28 days old)
SD	**Contact lens associated microbial keratitis** (*red eye, severe pain, photosensitive, visible ulcer*)
CM	**Corneal abrasion**: prescribe chloramphenicol ointment but *refer same day if trauma involved chemical or organic matter, or visible ulcer*
48h	**Corneal abrasion**: if not responding to treatment with no evidence of an ulcer
SSC	**Corneal dystrophies** (e.g. keratoconus)
24h	**Corneal foreign body if in stroma / rust ring or sub-tarsal foreign body**: prescribe chloramphenicol ointment until review
IR	**Endophthalmitis** (*post-op <2 weeks with severe pain / reduced vision / discharge*)
CM	**Episcleritis** (*sectoral redness with irritation*): advise lubricating eye drops and over-the-counter non-steroidal anti-inflammatory drugs (NSAIDs); reassure patient it self-resolves. Refer to ophthalmology if it does not resolve within 2–4 weeks
CM	**Facial nerve palsy**: normally investigated by GP / A&E / ENT; assess ability to close lid; suggest aggressive lubricating eye drops and/or ointment day and night, and tape eyelids at night; oculoplastics referral if lid closure remains poor; *refer same day referral to ophthalmology if patient develops red, painful eye (exposure keratopathy)*
24h	**Flashes and floaters**: all patients with new onset of symptoms especially high risk (i.e. myope, previous ocular surgery or trauma, previous or family history of retinal tear / detachment)
SD	**Flashes and floaters with new onset visual field defect**
SD	**Giant cell arteritis:** refer to ophthalmology if with ocular symptoms; refer to medics / rheumatology if no ocular symptoms. If urgent FBC, ESR, CRP obtained in community and suspicion is high, commence corticosteroids and then refer the same day

48h	**Herpes simplex keratitis** (*periocular rash with red/sore eye, dendrite*)
48h	**Herpes zoster** (*shingles rash to forehead ± red/sore eye, pseudodendrite*): prescribe oral antivirals and lubricating eye drops; and only refer to ophthalmology if associated with a red, painful eye
SD	**Hyphaema**
FTC	**Leucocoria or absent red reflex in a child**: discuss with the paediatric ophthalmology team for sooner review if there are other concerning features
SD	**Lid laceration**
SSC	**Lid malposition** (*with associated ocular irritation, recurrent conjunctivitis, keratopathy*): prescribe lubricating eye drops
SSC	**Macular hole**
48h	**Marginal keratitis:** known with symptoms for >48 hours
24h	**Marginal keratitis:** suspected; if new or unsure of diagnosis
SD	**Non-accidental injury** in a child
IR	**Orbital cellulitis** (*systemically unwell, reduced vision, diplopia, restricted eye movements, unable to open eye, relative afferent pupillary defect*): children must be referred directly to paediatric team
IR	**Severely painful eye following cataract surgery / intravitreal injection** in last 2–8 weeks especially if lid swelling, discharge, reduced vision
24h	**Papilloedema** (*bilateral disc swelling with symptoms suggestive of raised intracranial pressure (ICP)*): if confident of diagnosis, refer directly to medics; if unsure of diagnosis with symptoms suggestive of raised ICP, refer to ophthalmology for dilated fundoscopy to assess optic discs
IR	**Penetrating injury or intraocular foreign body** (*reduced vision, irregular pupil, shallow anterior chamber, hyphaema*): requires same day CT scan to assess for intraocular foreign body / globe rupture
CM	**Pinguecula**: prescribe lubricating eye drops
FTC	**Proptosis** (*gradual with no vision loss*)
SD	**Proptosis** (*pulsating or sudden onset with or without vision loss*)
FTC	**Retinal vein occlusion** with macular oedema
IR	**Retrobulbar haemorrhage** (*marked lid swelling and proptosis with reduced vision, unreactive pupil, restriction of eye movements + history of trauma*): refer for lateral canthotomy + cantholysis ± emergency imaging
48h	**Scleritis** (*severely red eye with toothache-like boring pain and underlying rheumatological condition*)
CM	**Subconjunctival haemorrhage**: spontaneous, no significant trauma, check BP, review medications (check international normalized ratio (INR) if on warfarin), reassure for self-resolution
SD	**Subconjunctival haemorrhage**: associated with trauma

SD	**Thyroid disease or thyroid eye disease** (*previously diagnosed disease with new acute vision loss or pain*)
24h	**Uveitis** (*red, sore, photosensitive eye with no surface / corneal pathology, especially if previous flares*)
CM	**Viral conjunctivitis** (*puffy red eyes with lid swelling, especially if recent respiratory tract infection*): cool compresses, lubricating eye drops, hygiene, reassure self-resolution within 2–4 weeks
48h	**Viral conjunctivitis with pseudomembranes**
24h	**Vitreous haemorrhage** (*sudden shower of dark / red–brown floaters and foggy vision*)
SD	**Wound infection in post-op patients**

Chapter 7
The orbit

7.1 Introduction

The orbit, or bony casing of the eye, was anatomically described in *Section 2.3*.

Orbital conditions can be notoriously difficult to diagnose and treat; however, they can be both sight- and life-threatening. Therefore, it is vital to have a sound system for assessing orbital presentations.

In this chapter, a systematic approach to recognizing and assessing an 'orbital' patient is provided, including clues as to what the likely diagnosis may be, and how to investigate, manage or refer such cases.

 The history, examination and initial investigations are usually done by the referrer, i.e. GP or A&E. Some conditions require immediate referral to ophthalmology, but others can be referred routinely.

The most common orbital conditions are:
- Thyroid orbitopathy
- Traumatic conditions (such as orbital fracture and retrobulbar haemorrhage)
- Orbital cellulitis (which can be life- and sight-threatening)
- Inflammatory conditions (myositis, idiopathic orbital inflammation)
- Vascular conditions (carotid-cavernous fistula)
- Tumours.

CLINICAL CONTEXT TIPS

What questions should be asked about someone with suspected orbital disease?

When taking the history it is vital to rule each of these in/out by asking about the following:
- Any known abnormal thyroid function tests or symptoms to suggest dysthyroidism?
  - *think thyroid eye disease*
- Any cardiovascular risk factors?
  - *think carotid-cavernous fistula*
- Any recent dental work, concurrent respiratory tract / sinus infections, fevers or systemically unwell?
  - *think cavernous sinus thrombosis or orbital cellulitis*
- Any preceding trauma?
  - *think retrobulbar haemorrhage*
- Any personal or family history of neoplasm?
  - *think lymphoma or metastasis*

7.2 What might an orbital condition look like?

Different causes of orbital pathology may have similar-looking presentations, so it is important to:
- Recognize the signs
- Consider and document the consequent symptoms
- Investigate thoroughly, but pertinently, in order to guide appropriate treatment.

Although we usually take an approach of history followed by examination, for the assessment of orbital conditions it can be useful to assess the pathological signs first, then think about what symptoms these may cause.

7.2.1 Signs and consequent symptoms

The following are signs and symptoms that may point towards orbital pathology, and which can be explored in both ophthalmic and non-ophthalmic settings. Reference is made to the relevant section for examination technique for each component:
- Resting position of lids
  - are the superior or inferior sclera visualized? (*Figure 7.1A*)
  - is there ptosis or pseudoptosis?
- Reduced visual acuity (blurred vision; see *Section 2.2*)
- Reduced colour vision (see *Section 2.2*)
- Abnormal visual field (see *Section 14.2*)
- Abnormal pupillary responses (is there a relative afferent pupillary defect?; see *Figure 2.20*)
- Restricted ocular motility (diplopia / double vision; see *Section 2.4.5*)
- Proptosis (hallmark of orbital pathology; see *Section 2.3*):
  - axial proptosis (see *Figure 7.1*): globe displaced anteriorly, i.e. forwards
  - non-axial proptosis (dystopia; see *Figure 7.3*): globe displaced vertically or horizontally
  - pulsatile proptosis: globe pulsating on observation or palpation (see *Section 2.3* on how to palpate for this)
  - proptosis may only be demonstrated on a Valsalva manoeuvre or on bending forward
  - globe retropulsion: resistance to reducing globe back into the orbit (see *Section 2.3* on the technique)
- Incomplete lid closure (lagophthalmos)
- Enophthalmos (globe displaced backward)
- Exposure keratopathy causing injected eye with photosensitivity and foreign body sensation.

Table 7.1 illustrates the different types of proptosis and the diseases that cause these different types.

Table 7.1 Proptosis features and associated disease

Proptosis feature	Disease
Axial	Thyroid eye disease
	Intraconal lesion (e.g. optic nerve glioma)
Dystopia	Dermoid
	Sinus disease
	Lacrimal gland tumour
Pulsatile	Carotid-cavernous fistula
	Sphenoid wing dysplasia secondary to neurofibromatosis I
	Orbital arteriovenous malformation
	Orbital roof fractures
Increased proptosis on Valsalva manoeuvre or bending forward	Orbital lymphaticovenous malformations
	Orbital varices

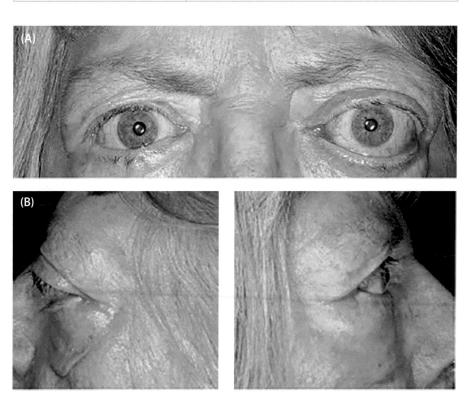

Figure 7.1 (A) Left-sided axial proptosis conjunctival injection and inferior scleral show. Cornea looks clear and pupils equal. (B) Lateral view of proptosis (left image).

There are a number of signs that may only be apparent on further
examination by the ophthalmologist:
- Formal documentation of proptosis or enophthalmos as measured with an
  exophthalmeter
- Assessing cornea and conjunctiva with sodium fluorescein 2% for evidence
  of exposure keratitis
- Braley's sign: increased intraocular pressure by more than 6mmHg in
  upgaze
  - *think thyroid eye disease* (enlarged inferior rectus blocking episcleral
    outflow in thyroid eye disease)
- Dilated fundus examination looking for:
  - optic disc swelling or atrophy
  - optociliary shunt vessels (also known as disc collaterals)
  - choroidal folds
    - due to external compression of the globe.

CLINICAL CONTEXT TIPS

What are optociliary shunt vessels?
Optociliary shunt vessels can be differentiated from new vessels at the disc
by their larger calibre and lack of leakage on angiography. They are caused by
ischaemic retinal conditions, chronic glaucoma and orbital conditions.

7.3 What are the causes of an orbital presentation?

Orbital pathology can have various causes and a 'surgical sieve' approach is a helpful
way to categorize them. *Table 7.2* details the different aetiologies of orbital disease.
Based on the results of this, you can then investigate to rule each one in or out.

7.3.1 Investigations

Initial investigations to further differentiate the cause would include:
- Vital signs including BP
- BG
- Blood tests
  - FBC
  - function tests:
    - kidney
    - liver
    - thyroid (with thyroid peroxidase antibodies)
  - inflammatory markers (CRP and ESR)
  - autoimmune screen
- Imaging
  - urgent CT head and orbit

Table 7.2 Aetiology of orbital disease

Aetiology	Disease
Acquired	
Vascular	Capillary or cavernous haemangioma
	Carotid-cavernous fistula (see *Section 7.4.4*)
	Cavernous sinus thrombosis (see *Section 14.6.2*)
	Orbital lymphaticovenous malformation
Inflammatory / infective	Orbital cellulitis (see *Section 7.4.2*)
Trauma	Retrobulbar haemorrhage (see *Section 7.4.1*)
Endocrine	Thyroid orbitopathy (the most common cause of proptosis; see *Section 7.4.3*)
Idiopathic	Idiopathic orbital inflammatory disease
Neoplastic	Lacrimal gland mass
	Lymphoma
	Sphenoid wing meningioma
	Optic nerve glioma
	Orbital metastases
	Rhabdomyosarcoma
Congenital	Orbital dermoid
	Craniofacial anomalies

○ magnetic resonance imaging (MRI) with contrast: further soft tissue detail is required (to assess the extent of orbitopathy and rule out mass lesions).

 In the ophthalmology clinic the following additional investigations should also be performed:
- Visual field testing
- Fundus photos
- Optical coherence tomography (OCT):
  ○ optic nerve (*think optic disc swelling or atrophy*)
  ○ macula (*think choroidal folds*).

With history, examination and investigations completed, patients with orbital disease should be referred to an ophthalmologist as follows:
- Immediate referral:
  ○ orbital cellulitis
  ○ severe thyroid eye disease
  ○ retrobulbar haemorrhage
- Same day:
  ○ pulsating proptosis
  ○ sudden onset proptosis with or without vision loss

○ sudden enophthalmos after trauma
- Fast-track clinic:
  ○ gradual proptosis with no vision loss
  ○ gradual enophthalmos with no vision loss.

CLINICAL CONTEXT TIPS

When should an 'orbital' patient with vision loss be seen?
There is always that clinical conundrum when a patient presents with a chronic history of proptosis or other globe displacement, but only seeks medical attention when there are perceived vision changes. As a general rule, vision loss should signal **same day referral**, as emergent management may prevent further vision loss or allow some visual function recovery. In patients with no vision loss and gradual globe displacement, always safety-net and ensure the patient reports if they do not get an appointment or if there are any vision changes.

The role of the ophthalmologist in these cases is to help identify the cause, assess the impact of orbital disease on the globe and visual function, treat ocular complications such as exposure keratitis, and follow up these patients as part of a multidisciplinary team (MDT). Members of the MDT include:
- Paediatrician: for any child with orbital signs
- Endocrinologist: if thyroid dysfunction is found
- Maxillofacial team: for orbital floor fractures
- Ear, nose and throat (ENT): for orbital cellulitis
- Neurosurgeons: for carotid-cavernous fistula (alongside interventional radiology and/or medical team), intracranial neoplasms (alongside neurology / neuro-oncology)
- Oncology: orbital primary malignancy or metastases.

7.4 Orbital presentations you need to understand

7.4.1 Retrobulbar haemorrhage

RED FLAG

- Consider this if acute proptosis with trauma
- **Urgent** lateral canthotomy + cantholysis required.

One of the very few 'true' ophthalmic emergencies and a relatively simple timely intervention can save the patient from going irreversibly blind. You don't necessarily need to be an ophthalmologist to diagnose or initiate treatment.

It is vital to ascertain a history of trauma in any patient with acute proptosis and a possible retrobulbar haemorrhage, but also consider iatrogenic causes (post-surgery) and spontaneous bleeding from orbital mass lesions. Air from an orbital wall fracture can also cause acute proptosis, and requires rapid orbital decompression. Orbital decompression is key in these conditions as the orbit has a maximum volume, which if exceeded means the tissue pressure in a closed muscle compartment exceeds the perfusion pressure, impairing blood outflow and resulting in muscle, nerve and vascular ischaemia.

History
- Trauma
- Anticoagulation
- Recent orbital surgery.

Examination
Look for:
- Proptosis
- Eyelid swelling
- Ecchymosis
- Chemosis
- Anterior chamber shallowing or irregular pupil that may suggest globe rupture
- Reduced visual acuity
- Reduced colour vision
- Reduced extraocular movement
- In trauma cases, it is vital to ensure there are no further life-threatening injuries, or for instance an open globe injury on the other eye.

 Posterior segment examination may reveal venous congestion or retinal arterial occlusion. This should be performed after the emergent orbital decompression treatment.

Investigations
Do not investigate simply to diagnose retrobulbar haemorrhage; it is a clinical diagnosis and any delay in treatment will threaten the patient's vision.

These patients may subsequently undergo imaging (e.g. to rule out concomitant injuries or after initial treatment to help locate a haematoma or foreign body). If there is no history of trauma, MRI with angiography or venography can be performed to exclude vascular malformations.

Management
- Urgent lateral canthotomy and cantholysis within 2 hours (see *Box 7.1*).

In many departments orbital decompression is undertaken by A&E, maxillofacial and ENT clinicians, but a non-ophthalmologist should only perform a lateral canthotomy and cantholysis if suitably trained to do so. The on-call ophthalmologist should be contacted immediately if there is no one available to perform the procedure. Subsequent monitoring of the patient's visual function can occur after the procedure to assess recovery. Healing after a canthotomy and cantholysis is usually good, even without the need for formal repair.

If there is no improvement, other medical treatment options include mannitol and acetazolamide (with strict monitoring by the medical team), orbital septotomy or bony orbital decompression.

7.4.2 Orbital cellulitis

Orbital cellulitis can be sight- and life-threatening. The general conundrum is differentiating this from the more common preseptal cellulitis (*Table 7.3*). Preseptal

---

BOX 7.1: GUIDANCE FOR LATERAL CANTHOTOMY AND CANTHOLYSIS

1. Instil topical anaesthesia.
2. Prepare the area with sterile solution.
3. Use a 27-gauge needle to instil combined lignocaine + adrenaline to the skin and deep subcutaneous tissue.

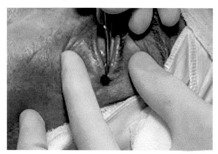

4. Using scissors (e.g. iris scissors) make a full thickness cut at the lateral canthus to create the canthotomy.

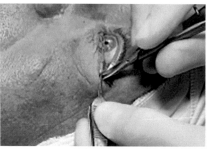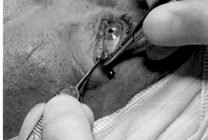

5. Using toothed forceps, pull the lower lid anteriorly (away from the globe) and cut the inferior (and, if possible, superior) crus of the tendon.
6. Post-procedure, apply chloramphenicol ointment to the wounds, but otherwise leave to heal naturally.
7. Assess for reduced proptosis, improved pupillary responses and improved visual function if patient is conscious.

Risks include: incomplete cantholysis, iatrogenic globe rupture or surrounding structure injury (rare), loss of adequate lower lid suspension and subsequent eyelid malpositioning, infection and bleeding.

---

cellulitis can be managed outside of ophthalmology (unless the diagnosis is uncertain), whereas orbital cellulitis needs emergency referral to the ophthalmology team as well as the adult or paediatric medical team.

To confirm preseptal cellulitis, you must have ensured that you have ruled out any signs or symptoms of orbital cellulitis (*Figure 7.2*).

Table 7.3 Differentiating between preseptal cellulitis and orbital cellulitis

	Preseptal cellulitis	**Orbital cellulitis**
History	Preceding trauma, bite, eyelid infection, e.g. stye Prior coryzal symptoms	Preceding adjacent structure infection, e.g. sinus disease, dental abscess, orbital surgery Upper respiratory tract infection Systemically unwell: fever, malaise Immunocompromised Visual symptoms: reduced vision or colour vision, diplopia or pain on eye movements
Examination	Afebrile or low grade fever No proptosis Mild eyelid swelling Normal visual acuity Normal pupillary reaction Normal colour vision	Febrile and systemically unwell Proptosis Grossly swollen eyelids Reduced visual acuity Relative afferent pupillary defect Reduced colour vision
	Signs of primary eyelid infection, e.g. hordeolum Normal extraocular movements 👁 Formal colour vision assessment if not available to referring clinician	Signs of primary eyelid infection less likely Restricted, painful extraocular movements 👁 Dilated fundus exam to look for optic disc swelling and choroidal folds Assessment of cornea to look for exposure keratopathy
Investigations	Mild disease: none Severe disease or unsure if orbital/sinus involvement: **refer immediately** for orbital cellulitis treatment protocol	Vital signs determine septic shock Urgent blood tests (FBC, CRP, blood cultures) Urgent CT orbit/sinus/brain with contrast (consider CT venogram if concerned for cavernous sinus thrombosis)

Table 7.3 *cont'd*

	Preseptal cellulitis	**Orbital cellulitis**
Management	Oral broad-spectrum antibiotics as per local guidelines	**Refer immediately for admission** and liaison with paediatric / adult medical team
	Cool compresses	Systemic resuscitation
	Analgesia	Intravenous antibiotics
	Strict safety-netting for progression	Discuss with orbital / ENT team regarding surgical intervention
	Regular clinical review	Daily ophthalmology review to monitor improvement
	NOTE	Switch to oral antibiotics with clinical improvement
	Paediatric patient with impaired eye opening:	
	refer immediately to ophthalmology + paediatric / adult medical team for admission and management	
	Treat as orbital cellulitis with orbital cellulitis treatment protocol	
	Switch to oral antibiotics with clinical improvement	

RED FLAG

Check for 'orbital signs' in any patient with preseptal cellulitis:
- Systemically unwell
- Proptosis
- Extraocular muscle movement restriction
- Chemosis
- Altered pupillary responses
- Reduced vision
- Optic disc swelling
- Choroidal folds.

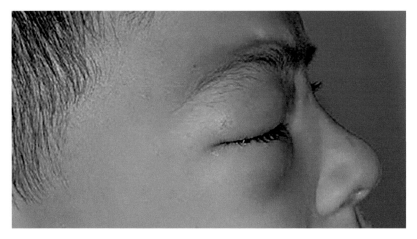

Figure 7.2 Orbital cellulitis: right-sided upper and lower lid erythematous swelling causing complete mechanical ptosis.

RED FLAG

In a systemically well child with acute or subacute proptosis ± dystopia, rhabdomyosarcoma should be on your differential diagnosis list as it can mimic orbital cellulitis (*Figure 7.3*).

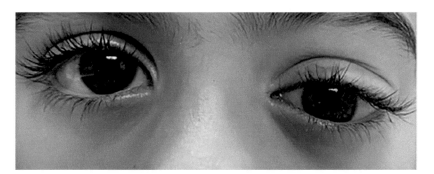

Figure 7.3 Left dystopia in suspected rhabdomyosarcoma.

7.4.3 Thyroid eye disease

Thyroid eye disease (TED) is the most common cause of unilateral and bilateral proptosis. It occurs when antibodies formed against the thyroid gland also attack the orbital tissues, resulting in inflammation of the extraocular muscles and orbital tissues. The extraocular muscles enlarge (initially inferior rectus, followed by medial rectus, superior rectus and lateral rectus) and cause axial proptosis. It is self-limiting, characterized by an active phase, with increasing disease severity, and an inactive phase. Although the majority of patients with TED are hyperthyroid, a proportion of patients may also be hypothyroid or euthyroid. Patients with TED can be referred to ophthalmology during the active or inactive phase.

Patients with thyroid dysfunction (past or present) presenting with orbital signs should be suspected of having TED. Blood tests, such as thyroid function tests and thyroid antibodies, can be useful for making the diagnosis.

RED FLAG

Patients with active disease with orbital signs, evidence of thyroid optic neuropathy and severe exposure keratopathy require an **urgent referral to ophthalmology** for medical and/or surgical management.

History

In addition to asking about signs and symptoms (see *Section 7.2.1*), in the ophthalmology setting the history should include:
- Date of thyroid dysfunction diagnosis (if not previously diagnosed, and there is clinical suspicion for TED, perform thyroid function tests and thyroid antibodies screen)
- Endocrine treatment history
- Past medical history
- Drug history
- Smoking status (smoking is a major risk factor for thyroid eye disease)
- Social history should include mood status and support, because thyroid eye disease can considerably affect quality of life.

The following thyroid eye disease symptoms should be documented:
- Gritty / dry / uncomfortable eyes
- Watery eyes
- Photosensitivity
- Subjective forward protrusion of the eye
- Reduced vision
- Diplopia.

Examination
Observe for:
- External eye appearance (*Figure 7.4*)
  - lid swelling and redness
  - conjunctival redness and swelling (chemosis)
  - proptosis
  - orbital firmness
  - lid retraction
    - superior scleral show
    - temporal flare: lid retraction more obvious lateral eyelid

- Restricted ocular motility
- Anterior segment inflammation
  - red eyes
  - chemosis
  - caruncle oedema (does the caruncle bulge through the lids with eyelid closure?)
- Lagophthalmos
- Exposure keratopathy
- Optic disc oedema
- Choroidal folds.

Test for lid lag (on dynamic testing, asking the patient to look down reveals a 'lag' in the downward movement of the upper lid).

CLINICAL CONTEXT TIPS

Grading of thyroid eye disease
Grading of thyroid eye disease is very useful in determining active vs. stable disease. It assesses both of the following:

- Severity (graded by amount of upper eyelid retraction, lid lag, eyelid and conjunctival swelling and redness, proptosis, ocular motility restriction, corneal involvement secondary to lagophthalmos and dysthyroid optic neuropathy effect on daily living)
- Activity (graded by ocular pain at rest or with eye movement, eyelid swelling and redness, conjunctival redness and chemosis, caruncle oedema, increase in proptosis, ocular motility restriction, change in visual acuity).

Various scoring systems exist for each and the most commonly used are:

- VISA (vision, inflammation, strabismus and appearance) score for both severity and activity
- European Group of Graves' Orbitopathy (EUGOGO) score for severity
- Clinical Activity Score (CAS) for activity.

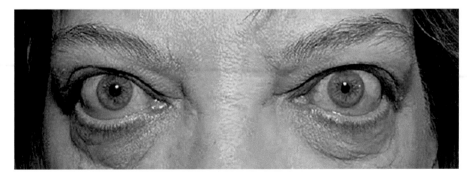

Figure 7.4 Bilateral proptosis with lid retraction, temporal flare and inferior scleral show.

Investigations

 Thyroid function tests are usually initiated and monitored by the GP and/or endocrinologist.

 An ophthalmologist should note the latest thyroid function tests, specifically thyroid-stimulating immunoglobulin and thyroid-stimulating hormone (TSH) receptor antibodies, which have been shown to be associated with thyroid eye disease. Ophthalmic investigations include visual field testing to rule out optic nerve functional deficit and, in some units, Hess chart to plot extraocular muscle movements. MRI imaging (T2 sequences with STIR (short tau inversion recovery)) classically is important, as it shows extraocular muscle enlargement with sparing of tendons.

Management

- MDT management
  - oculoplastics
  - strabismus
  - endocrinology / GP
- Systemic
  - optimize thyroid function (with the assistance of endocrinology and/or GP colleagues)
- Ocular
  - protect the cornea and optic nerve, with visual, ocular motility and oculoplastic rehabilitation
- Smoking cessation advice if appropriate
- Mild thyroid eye disease (mild symptoms and soft tissue changes, not impacting activities of daily living enough to justify immunosuppression):
  - conservative treatment with prisms / occlusion for diplopia, lubricating eye drops for the ocular surface and selenium supplementation
- Moderate thyroid eye disease:
  - weekly steroid therapy in accordance with local protocols. EUGOGO suggest 500mg intravenous methylprednisolone weekly for 6 weeks followed by 250mg weekly for 6 weeks with an increased recognition for the role of immunosuppression
- Sight-threatening thyroid eye disease (signs of compressive optic neuropathy or corneal breakdown / ulceration):
  - urgent admission of patients
  - co-management with medical and endocrinology teams
  - pulsed IV methylprednisolone (e.g. 1g as a single dose, repeated over 3 days) and daily monitoring
  - poor responders to high dose corticosteroids should be considered for urgent surgical decompression.

Patients can have orbital and lid changes that remain long after the acute inflammation has resolved due to fibrotic changes. In the long term, and once active disease has subsided, orbital decompression, strabismus and lid surgery (in that sequence) can be considered.

7.4.4 Carotid-cavernous fistula

Orbital presentation with tortuous 'corkscrew'-like episcleral blood vessels and pulsatile proptosis with an audible bruit should raise suspicion for carotid-cavernous fistula (CCF). A CCF is an abnormal communication between the carotid arterial and cavernous sinus venous circulation. They are classified as direct or indirect. Risk factors include trauma, hypertension and connective tissue disease.

History
Patients complain of pulsatile tinnitus and headache, and in more severe cases, diplopia and visual loss. Ask about:
- Trauma, including recent intracranial surgery (*think direct CCF; acute onset*)
- Connective tissue disease (*think indirect CCF; insidious onset*)
- Cardiovascular disease (*think indirect CCF*).

Examination
Observe for:
- Pulsatile proptosis
- Ptosis
- Tortuous 'corkscrew'-like episcleral blood vessels
- Eyelid oedema
- Ocular motility restriction
- Anisocoria.

In ophthalmic clinic other elements of examination include:
- Intraocular pressure
- Gonioscopy to detect blood in Schlemm's canal, indicating raised episcleral venous pressure
- Ocular motility assessment
- Cranial nerve palsy assessment
- Testing for Horner's syndrome with apraclonidine 1% (see *Section 14.7*)
- Dilated fundus exam looking for optic disc swelling, dilated retinal veins, retinal vein occlusion or choroidal detachment.

Investigation
- Urgent neuroimaging (CT or MRI with angiography) via **direct referral to A&E, medics or neurosurgical team**
- Gold standard imaging is with digital subtraction angiography.

Management
This is in collaboration with neurosurgeons, and can include observation for low flow indirect shunts or endovascular treatment for direct shunts (urgently in severe cases).

Ophthalmology input is required in the acute phase for conservative management of diplopia and raised intraocular pressure. Follow this with a collaborative approach with ophthalmology monitoring and treatment of any visual dysfunction, changes in intraocular pressure, ptosis and strabismus.

7.4.5 Enophthalmos

Although uncommon, enophthalmos (posterior displacement of the globe) can be a sign of serious disease, the causes of which are listed in *Table 7.4*.

Table 7.4 Causes of enophthalmos

Trauma	Orbital floor fracture
Neoplasm	Orbital metastases, e.g. from breast cancer (tumour growth and fibrosis leading to atrophy of retrobulbar fat, shrinkage of connective tissue)
Inflammatory	Silent sinus syndrome; where a 'vacuum effect' is caused due to disrupted maxillary sinus drainage
Age-related	Senile orbital fat atrophy
Iatrogenic	Prostaglandin analogue induced orbitopathy, radiotherapy
'Pseudo-enophthalmos'	Contralateral proptosis, Horner's syndrome, phthisis, ptosis, post-enucleation socket syndrome in artificial eye patients

In the pre-ophthalmology setting, the aim of clinicians is to ascertain how soon the patient with enophthalmos needs to be referred. A thorough history should help this decision-making, and as a general rule, any enophthalmos as a result of acute trauma or with vision dysfunction should have a **same day referral** to local eye services.

History
Ask about:
- Diplopia
- Change in facial appearance
- Pain
- Previous trauma
- History of malignancy (personal or familial).

Examination
Observe for:
- Eyelid changes (swelling, redness)
- Obvious orbital masses (see *Figure 2.2*)
- Globe displacement
- Ocular motility restriction
- Conjunctival redness or chemosis
- Pupillary changes
- Vision dysfunction.

In the ophthalmology department, further examination and tests include:
- Exophthalmometry
- Intraocular pressure
- Dilated fundus examination (looking for choroidal folds)

- Visual field
- OCT disc and macula.

Investigations
- CT orbital and facial imaging ± MRI (urgency depends on clinical course)
- Blood tests to rule out malignancy and inflammatory disease.

Management
This is guided by the underlying pathology and may require a multidisciplinary approach.

7.4.6 Anophthalmia

Anophthalmia, or absence of the eye(s) can be congenital or acquired.

Congenital anophthalmia requires the multidisciplinary input from oculoplastics, paediatric ophthalmology and low vision specialists.

Acquired anophthalmia is as a result of eye removal, the indications for which include:
- Malignancy (retinoblastoma, choroidal melanoma)
- Painful or cosmetically unacceptable phthiscal (a small, non-functional blind eye)
- Severe trauma, to prevent sympathetic ophthalmia (inflammation of the fellow eye following insult to the offending eye)
- Untreatable intraocular infection with severe endophthalmitis (purulent infection of the aqueous and/or vitreous humour).

Surgical options for eye removal include:
- Evisceration: eye content removal, leaving the sclera and extraocular muscles intact
- Enucleation: eye removal including sclera, leaving the extraocular muscles intact
- Exenteration: removal of eye and parts of the orbit.

An implant (for volume) and a temporary conformer (holding the fornices open) are almost always placed in conjunction with eye removal surgery. Following post-operative healing of the socket, an artificial eye can be fitted by an ocularist (a specialist in eye prostheses).

CLINICAL CONTEXT TIPS

Treatment options for blind painful eyes
Consideration for treatment options for blind painful eyes should include the cause, level of vision and pain. Treatment options include:
- Observation (doing nothing)
- Conservative management with low dose steroids and atropine for comfort
- Contact lenses or scleral shell prosthesis for cosmesis
- Surgery.

Psychological support and monocular protection (glasses and avoidance of contact sports) to the fellow eye should always be offered.

There are a number of post-surgical problems that can occur as a result of eye removal:
- Discharge
  - primarily due to socket dryness
  - secondary causes include giant papillary conjunctivitis due to mechanical inflammation or irritation, infection or tumour recurrence
  - treatment includes regular prosthesis cleaning, lubricating eye drops, anti-allergy / anti-inflammatory drops for inflammation as necessary, and consideration of implant removal for infection (deep socket infection may not respond well to topical antibiotics)
- Post-enucleation socket syndrome
  - ptosis, superior sulcus hollowing, ectropion and lax lower lid
  - treatment:
    - volume deficiency: prosthesis modification or replacement, exchanging for a larger implant, injection of filler into the orbit or dermis fat grafts
    - eyelid position: lateral tarsal strip or levator resection
- Contracted socket
  - aetiology:
    - primary cicatricial changes
    - socket infection / inflammation
    - multiple surgeries
    - poor compliance with wearing prosthesis
    - ill-fitted prosthesis
  - treatment
    - surgical to reform the scarred fornix
- Orbital implant exposure or extrusion
  - risk factors
    - inadequate surgical closure
    - infection
    - inflammation
    - small socket
  - treatment
    - topical / oral antibiotics
    - observe for spontaneous healing
    - surgery (implant exchange or dermis fat graft).

References and further reading

CAS score: Mourits, M.P., Koornneef, L., Wiersinga, W.M. *et al.* (1989) Clinical criteria for the assessment of disease activity in Graves' ophthalmopathy: a novel approach. *Br J Ophthalmol*, **73(8):** 639–644. doi:10.1136/bjo.73.8.639

EUGOGO: Bartalena, L., Kahaly, G.J., Baldeschi, L. *et al.* (2021) The 2021 European Group on Graves' orbitopathy (EUGOGO) clinical practice guidelines for the medical management of Graves' orbitopathy. *Eur J Endocrinol*, **185(4):** G43–G67. doi:10.1530/EJE-21-0479

VISA score: Dolman, P.J. and Rootman, J. (2006) VISA classification for Graves orbitopathy. *Ophthalmic Plast Reconstr Surg*, **22(5):** 319–324. doi:10.1097/01.iop.0000235499.34867.85

Chapter 8
Lashes, lids and lacrimal apparatus

LASHES

The main function of the eyelashes is to serve as a protective barrier for the eyes. Eyelash complaints may seem trivial, but they are common and can leave patients with troublesome symptoms. Eyelash conditions can also cause damage to the ocular surface and, if left untreated, can lead to sight-threatening corneal damage. Therefore it is important to have an understanding of the assessment and diseases of the eyelashes.

8.1 Lash malposition

Trichiasis occurs when the lashes arise from their normal position, but are posteriorly directed (towards the front surface of the eye). The eyelid position is normal (compared to an entropion, or in-turning of the eyelid, which can subsequently cause the eyelashes to turn inwards, causing 'pseudotrichiasis').

Trichiasis can either be isolated or secondary to chronic eyelid inflammation, infection, previous trauma or surgery to the area, or certain medications such as prostaglandin analogue drops.

History
- Irritation
- Foreign body sensation
- Eye pain
- Red eye
- Watery eye
- Photosensitivity
- Vision changes (suggestive of corneal involvement)
- Rule out secondary causes (inflammation, infection, previous trauma, surgery, topical medications).

Examination

Observe for:
- Eyelid malposition (specifically entropion)
- Red eyes
- Does the cornea appear clear? (instil sodium fluorescein 2% and use a blue cobalt light if available; see *Figure 2.12*).

Slit lamp examination for:
- Cicatricial changes (scar formation)
- Keratitis.

Management

- Minimally symptomatic, with minimal conjunctival injection and cornea clear:
  - lubricating eye drops or ointment to protect cornea
- **Refer routinely** to ophthalmology if remains symptomatic.

- Treat underlying disease
- Treat any keratitis / corneal ulcer (see *Section 9.4*)
- Ocular surface protection: lubricating eye drops, consider bandage contact lens
- Lash removal: epilation (temporizing measure only)
- Lash destruction: referral to oculoplastic clinic for electrolysis, cryotherapy or lash excision surgery.

CLINICAL CONTEXT TIPS

What is distichiasis?

Distichiasis is a much rarer condition where there is an extra row of lashes (arising from an abnormal position). Very rarely, it can be associated with a genetic syndrome (lymphoedema–distichiasis syndrome). Treatment approaches are similar to those for trichiasis, but a definitive solution is surgery.

8.2 Blepharitis

Blepharitis is very common and encompasses a variety of conditions resulting in eyelid margin inflammation. The spectrum of blepharitis ranges from being observed incidentally on examination in clinic to incredibly symptomatic patients.

Blepharitis can be anterior, posterior or mixed. It can affect the eyelid margin only, the conjunctiva and eyelid (blepharoconjunctivitis) or, in more severe disease, the cornea (blepharokeratoconjunctivitis).

History

Suspect blepharitis in patients with:
- Burning and gritty sensation
- Mild redness
- Crusting of eyelashes in the morning
- Unless severe, vision should not be affected.

Examination

- Rule out associated conditions, e.g. facial rosacea
- Look for obvious chalazia (see *Section 8.6.2*) and styes (see *Section 8.6.3*)
- Look for eyelid redness
- Look for eye redness
- Assess if cornea is clear.

- Ensure there are no focal lesions (i.e. lid margin tumours masquerading as blepharitis)
- Examine for co-existing dry eye (evaporative, due to 'clogged' oil glands)
- Rule out keratitis / corneal ulcer.

Blepharitis falls into two categories:
- Anterior blepharitis
  - seborrhoeic or staphylococcal
  - more clinical signs on anterior lid margin (anterior to the grey line; see *Figure 2.4*)
  - collarettes / scales at lash base.
- Posterior blepharitis
  - more signs on posterior lid margin (posterior to the grey line; see *Figure 2.4*)
  - inflamed meibomian gland openings
  - pouting of glands with oil globules
  - foamy tear discharge.

Management

- Conservative management:
  - warm compresses (available commercially; apply for 10 minutes twice daily), combined with lid massage and cleaning of the eyelid
  - lubricating eye drops
  - environmental measures such as humidifiers
  - high omega-3 diet
- If no relief or worsening despite good long-term compliance with conservative management, or significantly symptomatic, **refer routinely** to ophthalmology (but always advise the patient to continue all measures until review in ophthalmology clinic)
- If any doubt as to whether there is keratitis / corneal ulcer (cornea not clear or appears vascularized), **refer urgently** to ophthalmology.

- If conservative measures fail, topical chloramphenicol ointment can be used to reduce the bacterial load in anterior blepharitis
- Topical steroid drops can also be trialled if there are significant refractory flares
- Oral tetracyclines can be used in both anterior and posterior blepharitis or rosacea-associated blepharitis
- Treat keratitis / corneal ulcer.

Patients require careful counselling so that they understand there is no 'magic cure' for blepharitis, and that the treatment goal is symptom management with long-term regular self-care.

LIDS

8.3 Lid malposition

8.3.1 Entropion

Entropion is a clinical sign which occurs with the lower eyelid. The lower eyelid turns inward, so the normal architecture of the lid margin is not visualized. Causes of entropion include:

- Involutional: age-related and most common
- Cicatricial: shortening of the posterior lamella due to scar formation
- Spastic: spasm of muscles leading to intermittent inward rolling of the lid margin
- Congenital (rare).

History

Ask about:

- Red eye
- Watery eye
- Foreign body sensation
- Visibly in-turned lower eyelid
- Visual symptoms (secondary to eyelash cornea touch causing corneal damage)
- Age of onset (*think involutional entropion*)
- For cicatricial aetiology ask about:
  - trauma (physical and chemical)
  - trachoma
  - ocular cicatricial pemphigoid (OCP)
  - Stevens–Johnson syndrome (SJS)
- For spastic aetiology, ask about intermittency of symptoms
- For mechanical aetiology, enquire about history of malignancy.

Examination

Observe for:

- Inward turning of eyelids (usually the lower eyelid; *Figure 8.1*)
- Spasm of eyelids or facial muscles
- Watery eye
- Conjunctival redness
- Whether cornea is clear

Observe for:

- Blepharospasm or hemifacial spasm
- Lash corneal touch
- Epiphora
- Conjunctival redness
- Keratopathy / keratitis / corneal ulcer
- Epiblepharon (an extra layer of skin on the lower eyelid causing pseudotrichiasis)
- Rule out secondary causes:

- o   mechanical cause in involutional entropion, and palpate around the lid for masses
- Involutional aetiology:
  - o   check for lid laxity:
    - ▪ 'snapback' test: pull the eyelid away from the globe, noting how many millimetres the eyelid can be distracted away from the globe (>5mm is abnormal) and whether the time it takes for the eyelid to 'snap back' into anatomically correct position (a longer time suggests laxity)
    - ▪ medial canthal tendon laxity: gently pull lower eyelid laterally, and >2mm of punctual movement from the medial canthus is abnormal
    - ▪ lateral canthal tendon laxity: gently pull the lower eyelid medially, and >2mm of movement of the lateral canthus suggests lateral canthal tendon laxity.
- Cicatricial aetiology:
  - o   shortening of the fornices
  - o   obliteration of the punctum
  - o   symblepharon (adhesion between bulbar and palpebral conjunctiva)
  - o   ankyloblepharon (adhesion between the edges of the upper and lower eyelids).

Management

- Lubricating eye drops or ointment
- Lid-taping (from just below the lashes to the upper cheek) to mechanically 'out-turn' the lid whilst awaiting more definitive treatment
- **Routine referral** to ophthalmology
- **Urgent referral** if history of SJS, chemical injury red eye, or cornea not clear.

- Ocular surface protection as above, with consideration of bandage contact lens
- Treat any keratopathy / keratitis / corneal ulcer
- Surgery:
  - o   referral to oculoplastics team for lid-shortening procedures for horizontal laxity, or everting sutures / retractor plication for inferior retractor dehiscence

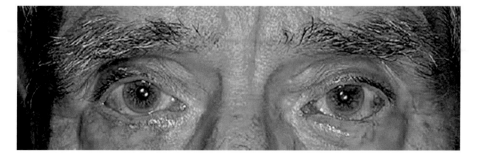

Figure 8.1 Left lower lid entropion with conjunctival hyperaemia. Cornea looks clear in this photo.

- Cicatricial disease is difficult to treat and requires an MDT approach to control the underlying process.

8.3.2 Ectropion

Ectropion is a clinical sign which usually occurs with the lower eyelid. The lower eyelid turns outward, so posterior to the meibomian gland openings and tarsal conjunctiva is visualized. Aetiology of ectropion is similar to entropion and includes:
- Involutional (common and usually age-related)
- Cicatricial
- Paralytic
- Congenital (rare)
- Mechanical (eyelid or cheek masses).

History
Ask about:
- Red eye
- Watery eye
- Foreign body sensation
- Visibly out-turned lower eyelid
- Inability to close eye fully
- Age of onset (*think involutional ectropion*)
- For cicatricial aetiology ask about:
  - trauma (physical and chemical)
  - previous eyelid or maxillary area surgery
  - dermatitis
  - radiotherapy
- For paralytic aetiology ask about Bell's palsy diagnosis or stroke
- For mechanical aetiology, enquire about history of malignancy.

Examination

Observe for:
- A visibly outward turning of the lower lid (*Figure 8.2*).
- Conjunctival redness
- Watery eye
- Is the cornea clear?
- Is the patient able to fully close their eye?
- Facial asymmetry.

- Facial features:
  - scarring, masses
  - facial asymmetry / evidence of facial nerve palsy
  - syndromic features
- Lid laxity as per entropion (see *Section 8.3.1*)
- Lagophthalmos
- Epiphora
- Conjunctival redness
- Keratopathy / keratitis / corneal ulcer.

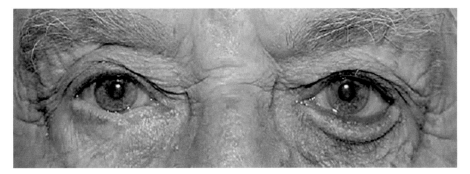

Figure 8.2 Left lower lid ectropion.

Management

- Lubricating eye drops or ointment
- Lid-taping (horizontally from the lower eyelid to the zygomatic region to hold lid up to a more correct anatomical position)
- **Routine** ophthalmology referral.

- Lubricating eye drops or ointment
- Treat keratopathy / keratitis / corneal ulcer
- Treat the underlying cause
- Surgery is definitive; referral to oculoplastics team for lid-shortening procedures for horizontal laxity.

8.3.3 Ptosis

Ptosis is also known as droopy eyelid, and mostly affects the upper eyelid. The main principles in evaluating ptosis (or a drooping lid) are:

1. Not every 'ptosis' is a ptosis; it is important to exclude causes of pseudoptosis (see *Clinical context tips* box below).
2. Ptosis is a sign, not a diagnosis; it is important to find the cause.
3. Some presentations of ptosis are sight- and/or life-threatening (although the majority are due to age-related / involutional changes).

Causes of true ptosis include (in descending order of life- / sight-threatening potential):

- Neurogenic
- Myasthenic
- Myogenic
- Congenital
- Mechanical
- Aponeurotic.

Box 8.1 highlights the various features of the different causes of true ptosis.

CLINICAL CONTEXT TIPS

What are the causes of pseudoptosis?

- Ipsilateral: brow ptosis, dermatochalasis (*Figure 8.3A*), phthisis or any cause of small / malpositioned globe (microphthalmos, prosthesis, enophthalmos)
- Contralateral: lid retraction, proptosis.

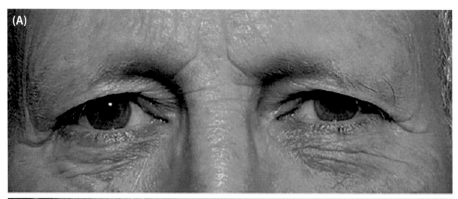

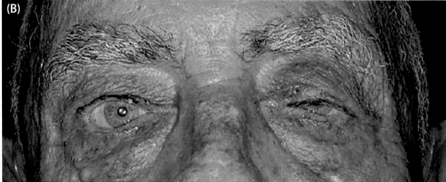

Figure 8.3 (A) Bilateral (left > right) dermatochalasis or excess upper lid skin, giving the appearance of 'pseudoptosis'. (B) Dermatochalasis and a true left-sided ptosis.

History

Ask about:

- Laterality
- Onset
- Duration (consider whether this is congenital, acute, subacute, post-surgical or chronic / long-standing)
- Visual disturbance (blurred vision, diplopia, visual field changes)
- Headache
- Fatigue
- Variability of ptosis (is it worse at the end of the day?)
- Problems with speech, breathing or swallowing
- Previous trauma (especially neck trauma)
- Previous ocular surgery
- Smoking status
- Systemic symptoms
- Family history of ptosis
- Effect on quality of life.

RED FLAG

Patients presenting to any clinical setting with acute-onset ptosis must have a fairly in-depth history and examination, as the signs and symptoms will determine where it is most appropriate to refer the patient. Not all patients with ptosis should be referred to ophthalmology first and it is vital to have a handle on whether this is an acute emergent ptosis (e.g. Horner's syndrome, third nerve palsy) or a chronic ptosis.

BOX 8.1: CAUSES OF TRUE PTOSIS

Neurogenic

Third cranial nerve palsy

Clinical features:

- (Mostly) complete ptosis
- Eye in 'down and out position'
- Ocular motility restriction
- Pupil fixed and dilated (although not always)
- Headache
- Diplopia.

Causes:

- Posterior communicating artery aneurysm until proven otherwise.

Investigations:

- Emergent CT/MR angiogram if acute presentation
- Always scan independent of whether or not pupil is involved.

Management:

- Depending on cause
- Confirmed aneurysms need emergency neurosurgical input
- Ophthalmologist and orthoptist: conservative management with prisms if ptosis is not complete or recovering and patient experiences diplopia.

Horner's syndrome

Clinical features:

- Partial ptosis
- Miosis (smaller) affected pupil
- Anhidrosis on the affected side
- Iris heterochromia: difference in eye colour
- Headache.

Causes:

- Categorized by which level of the nervous system is affected:
  - first order (central; hypothalamus to spinal cord / ciliospinal centre of Budge): stroke, demyelination, neoplasms

---

- second order (preganglionic; spinal cord to superior cervical ganglion): Pancoast tumour, neck dissection
- third order (postganglionic; superior cervical ganglion to orbit): internal carotid artery dissection or cavernous sinus thrombosis.

Investigations:
- Emergent CT/MR angiogram including the head, neck and chest
- **Emergent referral** to ophthalmology if there is concern about diagnosis and for formal pupil check
  - apraclonidine 1% helps with diagnosis of Horner's syndrome (see *Section 14.7*).

Management:
- Depending on cause.

Myasthenic

Myasthenia gravis

Clinical features:
- Bilateral, asymmetrical and variable ptosis
- Variable diplopia
- Fatigue
- Speech and swallow symptoms
- Limb weakness.

Causes:
- Autoimmune condition due to post-synaptic acetylcholine receptor antibodies.

Investigations:
- Acetylcholine receptor antibodies
- Muscle-specific kinase (MuSK)
- Ice pack test: ice pack on ptotic lid for 2 minutes improves the ptosis by 2mm
- Electromyography
- CT chest to look for thymoma.

Management:
- MDT approach to treatment
- Neurology: medically manage symptoms with anticholinesterase inhibitors such as pyridostigmine or immunosuppression
- Counselling on life-threatening myasthenic crisis
- Ophthalmologist and orthoptists: to monitor symptoms and treat conservatively with prisms in the acute phase
- Surgery avoided due to unpredictability.

Myogenic (rare)

Clinical features:
- Bilateral, symmetrical ptosis with systemic features / family history.

Myotonic dystrophy:
- Muscle wasting

- Delayed relaxation of muscles that are able to contract
- Cataracts
- Heart conduction abnormalities
- Pulmonary failure.

Chronic progressive external ophthalmoplegia (CPEO):
- Ocular motility restriction (rarely complain of diplopia as is symmetrical)
- Expressionless face
- Hearing loss
- Cataracts
- As part of Kearns–Sayre syndrome: heart block, pigmentary retinopathy.

Causes:
- Myotonic dystrophy: genetic mutation *DMPK* gene (autosomal dominant)
- Chronic progressive external ophthalmoplegia: mitochondrial disorder.

Investigations:
- Myotonic dystrophy: genetic testing
- CPEO: muscle biopsy (ragged red fibres)
- Electrocardiogram (ECG) to assess for heart conduction disorders.

Management:
- Supportive
- Multidisciplinary
- Caution with general anaesthetic, as it can lead to respiratory failure for these patients
- Surgery avoided due to unpredictability.

Congenital
Clinical features:
- Absent lid crease in ptotic eyelid
- Sensory deprivation amblyopia (see *Section 1.4.1*).

Causes:
- Congenital levator dysgenesis (most likely)
- Other causes: neurogenic (Horner's, third cranial nerve palsy), birth trauma, periorbital tumour, Marcus Gunn jaw-winking syndrome).

Investigations:
- None needed unless there is concern for neurogenic causes.

Management:
- Mild cases: no surgical intervention
- Affecting visual axis: time-critical and MDT approach (paediatric ophthalmology and oculoplastic) is crucial to prevent amblyopia
- Surgery (frontalis sling).

Mechanical
Clinical features:
- Eyelid swelling and redness

- Palpable mass
- Ocular motility restriction, proptosis, pupil abnormality.

Causes:
- Eyelid masses
- Eyelid inflammation (e.g. orbital cellulitis, see *Section 7.4.2*).

Investigations:
- CT/MR orbits
- Biopsy if appropriate.

Management:
- Dependent on cause.

Aponeurotic (the most common and least 'worrisome' cause of ptosis)

Clinical features:
- Deep superior sulcus
- High skin crease
- Superior visual field obscuration.

Causes:
- Age-related changes
- Previous ocular surgery with eyelid speculum use.

Investigations:
- Visual field test to demonstrate superior field obscuration
- No imaging unless concern for worrying features (ocular motility restriction, pupil abnormality, palpable mass).

Management:
- Dependent on cause
- Surgery (strict counselling of patient required, given unpredictable results).

RED FLAG

All patients with ptosis should have an ocular motility examination to assess for any restriction, and check of pupils for asymmetry in size and responses.

Examination

- Observe for:
- Visibly droopy eyelid (partial or total)
- Do the eyes move appropriately?
- What is the eye position?
- Eyelid changes (redness or swelling)
- Pupil abnormality
- Vision changes.

- Abnormal head position (chin up)
- Frontalis muscle (forehead) overaction
- Facial asymmetry
- Vision (especially in children at risk of amblyopia)
- Pupil responses and asymmetry
- Ocular motility (see *Figure 2.9*)
- Change in eyelid position:
  - on extraocular muscle movements: regeneration suggestive of chronic traumatic or intracranial lesions compressing on the third cranial nerve
  - on chewing: Marcus Gunn jaw-winking syndrome
- Ptosis:
  - document partial or total
  - assess skin crease, sulcus depth, palpebral aperture, margin-to-reflex distance 1 and 2 (*Figure 8.4*), levator function (*Figure 8.5*), lid margin to brow distance
- Lid:
  - evert lid for masses
  - assess for lagophthalmos (eyelid closure)
  - orbicularis tone: ask the patient to squeeze eyes tight whilst you try to open the lid
  - Cogan's twitch (myasthenia): overshoot of eyelid on sudden return to primary position after period of downgaze

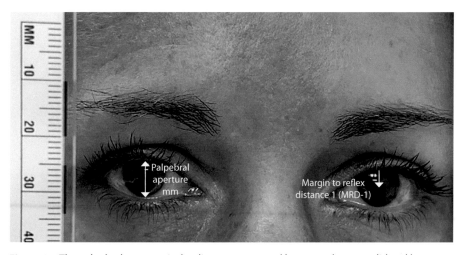

Figure 8.4 The palpebral aperture is the distance measured between the upper lid and lower lid margins with the eye open (it is usually around 10mm). The margin-to-reflex distance 1 is the distance measured between the upper lid margin and the corneal reflex at the centre of the pupil (usually around 3–4mm). The margin-to-reflex distance 2 is the remaining distance between the corneal reflex down to the lower lid margin (usually around 6mm).

- Assess cornea
  - ○ test sensation
  - ○ test Bell's phenomenon
- Assess for iris heterochromia.

Investigations
Dependent on the clinical context (see *Box 8.1*).

Management
- Dependent on aetiology
- Exclude pseudoptosis

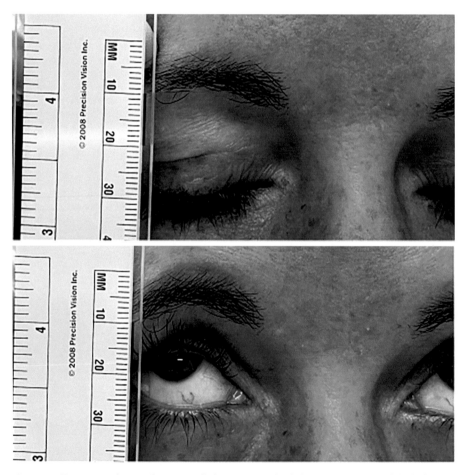

Figure 8.5 To measure levator function ask the patient to look down (top image) whilst holding your thumb against their forehead (occluding the effect of frontalis). Note the ruler marking at the upper lid lashline. Then ask the patient to look all the way up (bottom image). Note the new ruler marking where the upper lid lashline is now. The difference between the two measurements (excursion of upper eyelid) is the levator function.

- Surgical management is indicated for symptomatic ptosis and dependent on levator function
- Surgery is avoided in myogenic or myasthenic causes due to significant unpredictability of outcomes
- Refer routinely to the oculoplastic team (unless congenital and high risk of amblyopia)
- Surgical options depend on levator function and include conjunctivo-Müller resection, anterior levator resection, levator aponeurotic advancement, frontalis suspension with either autologous fascia lata or silicone slings.

8.4 Lid lumps

The main concern when assessing a lid lump is whether it is benign or malignant.

Having a clear system for assessment will enable accurate triage when referring to ophthalmology and will ensure you and your patient have peace of mind when assessing these lesions in clinic. Red flags for malignancy are marked in red.

History
Ask about:
- Onset and duration
- Change in size, shape or colour
- Bleeding, itching, ulceration or oozing
- Personal or family history of skin cancers
- Risk factors for skin cancer: age, occupational or recreational sun exposure, immunocompromise, smoking
- Medical and drug history (specifically genetic cancer syndromes and anticoagulants for surgical planning).

Examination

Observe for:
- Location – laterality, location on the lid, superficial or deep
  - basal cell carcinomas: more common on medial and lower lid
  - sebaceous gland carcinoma: more common on upper lid
  - fixation to the underlying bone
- Number of lesions (single, multiple)
- Pigmentation: what colour, homogeneous or heterogeneous
- Borders: distinct or indistinct
- Morphology: flat or elevated (nodular, papular, plaque, pustule, vesicular), ulceration and edges (rolled / pearly edges: basal cell carcinoma)
- Vascular features: telangiectasia is a hallmark for basal cell carcinoma
- Keratinization: a hallmark for squamous cell carcinoma
- Destructive features: distorting normal lid anatomy, loss of lashes
- Fixation to the underlying bone.

- Note skin colour: use Fitzpatrick scale
- Visual acuity

85

- Extraocular movements to rule out orbital involvement
- Syringing of lacrimal system if near this location
- Reduced eyelid sensation.

Management

- Refer routinely if no suspicious features, but refer on fast-track (2 week wait) pathway if there are any suspicious features
- Photo-documentation of the lesion for a baseline record and aid with triage is useful.

- Investigate with diagnostic biopsy (incision / excision) under oculoplastic team
- Imaging may be indicated for extensive tumours with potential orbital involvement
- Squamous cell carcinomas and malignant melanomas require an MDT approach from the investigation stage (including lymph node / whole-body imaging)
- Treatment is cause-dependent and will usually involve surgery for removal with margins if indicated
- Patients must be given sun protection advice.

8.5 Lid lesions – malignant

Malignant lid lesions may demonstrate significant change in size, shape or colour over time, and they may ulcerate, bleed, ooze or itch. Most lid malignancies are basal cell carcinomas (*Figure 8.6*), followed in frequency by squamous cell carcinomas and malignant melanoma (rare). The features and management of all are described in *Table 8.1*.

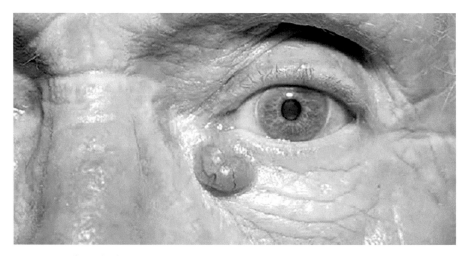

Figure 8.6 Left medial lower lid with single raised flesh-coloured lesion with rolled, pearly edges and telangiectasia suggestive of basal cell carcinoma.

Table 8.1 Features and management of lid malignancies

	Typical features	**Typical management**
Basal cell carcinoma	Superficial, nodular, infiltrative or sclerosing Commonly nodular with rolled, pearly edges, telangiectasia	Diagnostic incision biopsy followed by Mohs micrographic surgery (gold standard) or wide local excision with 2–3mm margins with histological control followed by reconstruction Other treatment modalities: topical imiquimod, photodynamic therapy (PDT) or cryotherapy for small / superficial lesions. In select cases radiotherapy is an option if not suitable for surgery. Local funding may be available for immunotherapy, e.g. vismodegib
Squamous cell carcinoma	Nodular hyperkeratotic lesion, cutaneous horn, ulceration Pre-malignant lesions such as actinic keratosis, Bowen's disease and keratoacanthoma can mimic squamous cell carcinoma and warrant diagnostic biopsy	Diagnostic incision biopsy Refer to cancer MDT to consider further scans and guide treatment (orbital CT, MRI, further body scans, lymph node investigation). Treatment is with Mohs or wide local excision with 5mm margins with histological control followed by reconstruction Orbital involvement may necessitate exenteration. Lymph node dissection may be required
Malignant melanoma	Darkly pigmented lesion; can be elevated (e.g. nodular) or flat (e.g. superficial spreading, lentigo malignant melanoma)	Diagnostic incision biopsy Refer to cancer MDT to consider further scans and guide treatment (orbital CT, MRI, further body scans, lymph node investigation) Treatment is with wide local excision with >10mm margins New immunomodulatory treatments have also been described. Lymph node dissection may be required

8.6 Lid lesions – benign

These lumps tend to be chronic and painless (except for acute inflammation in chalazia and styes) with no loss of lashes, destruction of lid anatomy, telangiectasia, ulceration or reduced sensation.

8.6.1 Eyelid cysts

These small spherical cystic nodular lesions represent blockages of apocrine ducts. A cyst of Moll is a translucent, clear fluid filled lesion due to a blockage of an apocrine duct (*Figure 8.7*). A cyst of Zeis is an opaque, yellow–white lesion due to a blockage in a sebaceous gland (*Figure 8.8*).

Management

Refer routinely to oculoplastic team if symptomatic and no suspicious features
Refer via fast-track clinic if suspicious features.

Can excise if patient symptomatic.

8.6.2 Chalazion

This is a sterile, chronic lipogranulomatous inflammation of a blocked meibomian gland (internal hordeola). This common condition (*Figure 8.9*) usually presents with a painless lump, though they can become either acutely inflamed or infected (internal hordeolum, which can discharge through the skin) as an erythematous, painful lesion with associated lid swelling. Inflamed blocked meibomian glands usually cause preseptal, and not orbital cellulitis (see *Section 7.4.2*).

Risk factors include blepharitis, seborrhoeic dermatitis and rosacea.

Management

- Encourage regular long-term warm compresses, lid massage, lid hygiene (see *Section 8.2*)
- Distinguish between preseptal and orbital cellulitis and treat with appropriate management of systemic ± topical antibiotics (see *Section 7.4.2*)
- If this fails or there is recurrent acute inflammation and the patient meets local criteria (e.g. wait 6 months for self-resolution prior to referral), **refer routinely** to ophthalmology for incision and curettage.

8.6.3 Stye

Stye and chalazia are often confused by both patients and clinicians, and it is sometimes difficult to clinically distinguish between them. Styes (external hordeola) represent an abscess within a lash follicle (usually due to *Staphylococcus* infection), and usually present acutely as a tender, small, localized erythematous elevated nodule with a yellow pus-filled head on the outer lid surface. There can be associated upper eyelid swelling and redness.

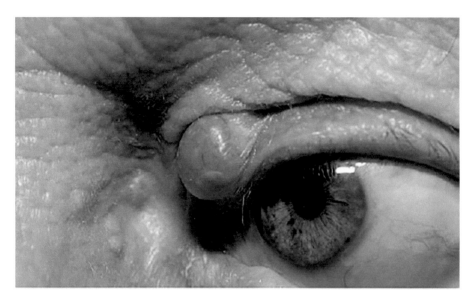

Figure 8.7 Left upper lid with medial translucent, fluid-filled cyst of Moll.

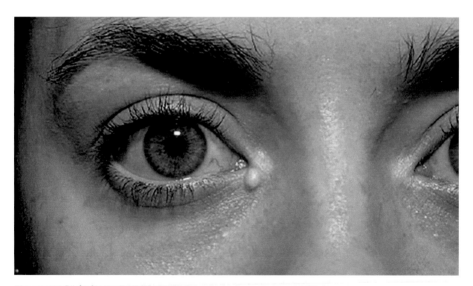

Figure 8.8 Right lower lid with medial canthal sebaceous cyst of Zeis.

Management

- Encourage regular long-term warm compresses, lid massage, lid hygiene (see *Section 8.2*)
- Acutely, encourage warm compresses and avoidance of make-up and contact lenses
- Most will resolve (or discharge spontaneously) within a week

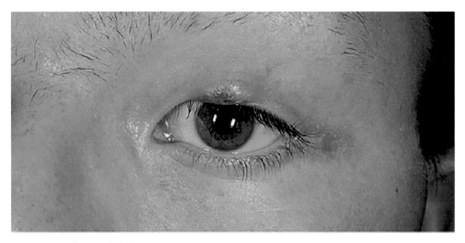

Figure 8.9 Left upper lid chalazion.

- Treat with topical chloramphenicol ointment
- Distinguish between preseptal and orbital cellulitis and treat with appropriate management of systemic + topical antibiotics (see *Section 7.4.2*).

LACRIMAL APPARATUS

8.7 Epiphora

'Watery eyes' or epiphora can be secondary to a variety of problems:
- Increased production: either increased basal production (rare) or, more commonly, reflex production, due to an ocular surface problem such as inflamed or dry ocular surface (most commonly: blepharitis and evaporative dry eye)
- Reduced drainage: due to lid position, such as ectropion (*Section 8.3.2*), blink-pump mechanism failure, such as in facial nerve palsy, or obstruction.

Obstruction can be at any level from the ocular surface to the nasolacrimal system and may be secondary to:
- Conjunctival chalasis: redundant folds of conjunctiva obscuring the punctum
- Punctal atresia or stenosis: a narrowed tear duct
- Canalicular or nasolacrimal duct obstruction: a blockage further down the tear drainage system
  - primary – idiopathic, usually involutional stenosis / fibrosis
  - secondary – endogenous inflammation, e.g. sarcoidosis, exogenous inflammation, e.g. chemical injury or burns, neoplasm, trauma or surgery, lacrimal stones, or displaced punctal plugs.

Most patients with epiphora will have an ocular surface problem and many of them can be managed without referral to ophthalmology. Rarely, patients may have lacrimal system malignancy where epiphora may be a presenting complaint.

History

Ask about:

- Laterality
- Duration
- Timing (constant indicates true nasolacrimal duct obstruction)
- Environmental factors: worse outdoors, in windy conditions or cold weather (worse indoors indicates more of a true nasolacrimal duct obstruction)
- Direction of tear flow: medially indicates punctal stenosis, laterally indicates lateral horizontal lid laxity
- Crusting of eyes in the morning (blepharitis), gritty (dry eye), itchy (atopy / allergic conjunctivitis)
- Haemolacria: blood in the tears is a hallmark for malignancy
- Past medical history and drug history (specifically: atopy, any nose trauma or surgery, inflammatory conditions or cancers, anticoagulant use for surgical planning).

Examination

- Rule out facial nerve palsy
- Assess eyelid position (ectropion / entropion)
- Assess eyelash position (trichiasis)
- Assess for blepharitis
- Grossly assess for any large masses in the lacrimal sac region
- Is the conjunctiva red?
- Is the cornea clear?

- Eyelid assessment (see *Section 8.3.1*)
- Press over lacrimal sac region for masses or any pus discharge (mucocele; see *Figure 8.10*)
- Is there evidence of dacryocystitis? (inflammation of the lacrimal sac)
- Check position of punctum (everted or stenosed?)
- Check conjunctival status with both lids everted (chalasis or inflammation?)
- Check tear meniscus height and quality of tears
- Treat keratopathy / keratitis / corneal ulcer
- Assess for anterior chamber inflammation
- Fluorescein dye disappearance test
  - assess time it takes for dye to disappear into nasolacrimal system
- Lacrimal syringing and probing with sterile saline
  - insert a sterile lacrimal cannula attached to a 2.5ml syringe filled with normal saline gently into the inferior punctum
  - insertion should be firstly vertical and then horizontal to follow the course of the canaliculi (see *Section 2.4.4*)
  - the findings of this test are:
    - anatomically patent system: a hard stop (cannula advances to the lacrimal sac and is abutting the lacrimal bone) and patency (patient tasting the saline solution on its injection) indicates an anatomically functioning system

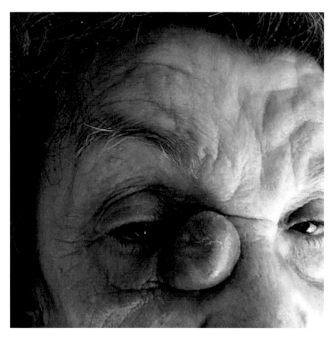

Figure 8.10 Mucocele of the right eye.

- canalicular obstruction: a soft stop (cannula does not advance to the lacrimal sac) with regurgitation on injection of the saline solution
- nasolacrimal duct obstruction: reflux through the superior puncta with mucus.

RED FLAG

Masses over the medial canthal area (without signs of infection) should be considered malignant until proven otherwise.

Investigations

Only needed for the minority of patients where there is clinical suspicion:
- Blood tests (*think underlying systemic inflammatory condition*)
- Imaging studies to delineate structure and function of lacrimal system (dacryocystography or dacryoscintigraphy) or CT/MRI to assess structure of lacrimal system with sinuses
- History of nasal trauma or surgery: refer to ENT team for nasal assessment.

Management

A large proportion of patients with epiphora will have conditions such as blepharitis, dry eye or allergic conjunctivitis, which can be safely managed without ophthalmology referral. Preservative-free lubricating eye drops, warm compresses, lid hygiene and massage, and over-the-counter anti-allergic drops where indicated, can be trialled. If consistent conservative measures do not help or if there is suggestion of further pathology (unilateral symptoms, history of nasal trauma or surgery, or obvious lid/lash malposition) a **routine referral** to ophthalmology is warranted. Masses or haemolacria warrant a **fast-track clinic referral**.

Dependent on cause and undertaken by the oculoplastic team.
- Conjunctival chalasis:
  - lubricating eye drops to improve tear lake
  - consideration of surgery if remains symptomatic
- Punctal stenosis:
  - punctal dilation for temporary relief
  - surgical punctoplasty for definitive treatment
- Dacryocystorhinostomy:
  - primary nasolacrimal duct obstruction
  - aim of surgery is to bypass part of the tear duct system by making a new connection from the lacrimal sac to the nasal cavity
- Secondary nasolacrimal duct obstruction is addressed by treating the cause.

Chapter 9

Conjunctiva, cornea and sclera

9.1 Introduction

The anatomy of the conjunctiva, cornea and sclera was discussed in *Sections 2.5* and *2.6*. There are a number of conditions that can affect these structures, particularly infection, inflammation and dry eyes. Some conditions that affect the cornea and sclera can be sight-threatening, and in the case of the sclera, can also be life-threatening if inflammation is secondary to a granulomatous necrotizing vasculitis such as granulomatosis with polyangiitis (GPA) (see *Chapter 21*).

9.2 Dry eye disease

Dry eye disease (DED) is most commonly due to an evaporative reason, owing to the tears not remaining on the surface of the eye for a sufficient amount of time. This is often due to poor oil layer (see *Section 2.4.3*) production, caused by conditions such as blepharitis (see *Section 8.2*). Systemic conditions such as Sjögren's disease and rheumatoid arthritis, as well as eyelid disease and malposition, previous trauma, surgery, systemic medications and contact lens wear, can all cause DED.

History
Ask about:
- Onset and duration
- Laterality
- Burning
- Itching
- Foreign body sensation
- Stringy discharge
- Eye redness
- Watery eye, especially in cold or windy weather
- Vision changes
- Triggering event (trauma or surgery)
- Eyelid malposition or poor closure
- Contact lens wear
- Any dry mouth, i.e. does the patient have a diagnosis of Sjögren's disease?
- Medications.

Examination

In-depth examination of the eyelids, cornea and conjunctiva requires the use of a slit lamp and fluorescein 2% (see *Figure 2.12*). The following is a schematic examination that can be performed in the ophthalmology setting to assess the tear film and ocular surface integrity:
- Eyelids

- is there crusting of the eyelids (blepharitis), frothy discharge at the eyelid margin or styes / chalazia (meibomian gland disease)?
- are the superior and inferior puncta patent?
- Instil fluorescein 2% and observe under the cobalt blue filter
  - what is the tear break-up time? (TBUT; time in seconds between a blink and when the first dry spot appears on the cornea – less than 10 is abnormal)
  - are there punctate epithelial erosions? (PEEs; small circular areas of fluorescein uptake)
- Schirmer's test
  - assessment of tear production.

Management

- Elimination of blepharitis and meibomian gland disease (see *Section 8.2*)
- Lubricating eye drops
- If still symptomatic despite strict compliance with conservative measures, a **routine referral** can be made to general eye ophthalmology or cornea service for further input
- Reiterate to the patient to continue using their lubricating eye drops until reviewed by the specialist.

- Punctal plugs (to stop the tears draining as quickly)
- Escalation of eye drop management (ciclosporin and autologous serum).

CLINICAL CONTEXT TIPS

Patient advice on lubricating eye drops
It is important to reiterate to patients with DED that lubricating eye drops need to be used at least four times a day, and can be used up to hourly if necessary.

9.3 Conjunctiva

9.3.1 Conjunctivitis

Conjunctivitis is inflammation of the conjunctiva. Patients presenting with conjunctivitis will have a variety of symptoms depending on the aetiology. *Table 9.1* gives a quick reference to the type of symptoms related to the main cause of conjunctivitis and can guide history and examination.

Management

Most cases of conjunctivitis are viral or allergic and can be managed in the community. However, the following exceptions apply and require **urgent referral** to ophthalmology:

- Contact lens wearer
- Trauma with organic matter

- Where the conjunctivitis does not resolve after a second course of topical treatment
- Neonate less than 28 days old (see *Section 15.3.3*).

- Persistent or recurrent conjunctivitis (the '2 and 2 rule': lasting more than 2 weeks or 2 courses of antibiotics): swabs should be taken for microscopy, culture and sensitivity, viral polymerase chain reaction (PCR), and chlamydia.
- Follow-up for patients with conjunctivitis can be a clinical judgement, and dependent on the microbiology results.

Table 9.1 Key signs and symptoms of different types of conjunctivitis (excluding neonatal conjunctivitis; see *Section 15.3.3*)

Aetiology	Symptoms	Signs	Treatment
Bacterial	Gritty sensation/pain Red eye Eyelashes stuck together Unilateral, occasionally bilateral	Lid swelling Green or yellow discharge (copious in gonococcal infection) Papillae ('red top')	Topical antibiotics Gonococcal aetiology: topical antibiotics plus systemic cephalosporin
Viral	Gritty sensation/pain Red eyes Unilateral but spreads to be bilateral Recent cold-like infection	Lid swelling Watery/'stringy' discharge Follicles ('white top'; *Figure 9.1*)	Artificial tears Cool compresses Herpes simplex aetiology: topical antivirals
Chlamydial	Gritty sensation Red eye Unilateral	Copious discharge Follicles (*Figure 9.1*)	Topical chloramphenicol Oral antibiotics (azithromycin or doxycycline)
Allergic	Itchy sensation Red eyes Swelling of eyelids Bilateral	Lid swelling Watery/mucoid discharge Papillae	**Mild**: artificial tears **Moderate**: mast cell stabilizer or topical antihistamine and oral antihistamine **Severe**: topical immunosuppressants

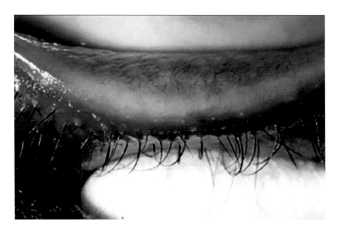

Figure 9.1 Follicular conjunctivitis: lymphoid hyperplasia with vascular base.

- Cornea specialist help should be sought early in cases which involve the cornea (corneal vascularization and opacification; *Figure 9.2*) or in older patients (>60 years) where there is concern for ocular mucous membrane pemphigoid with symblepharon formation (*Figure 9.3*).

CLINICAL CONTEXT TIPS

How to manage persistent conjunctivitis
Persistent unilateral conjunctivitis should raise the suspicion of chlamydial conjunctivitis (see *Table 9.1*). The patient should be counselled for the eventuality of a positive result, and the importance of systemic treatment should be stressed. It should even be considered in children with persistent unilateral infection, and parental discussion is key due to the safeguarding implications.

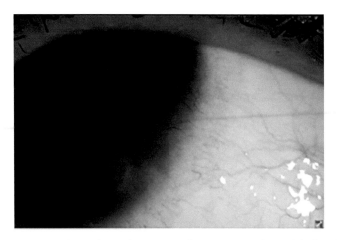

Figure 9.2 Corneal vascularization and opacity secondary to blepharokeratoconjunctivitis.

97

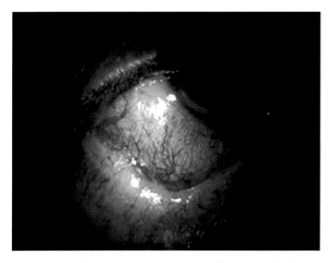

Figure 9.3 Symblepharon with shortening of the inferior fornix.

9.3.2 Conjunctival lesions

A number of lesions can involve the conjunctiva, and range from pigmented (e.g. a naevus; *Figure 9.4*) to non-pigmented (e.g. a pinguecula, *Figure 9.5* or a pterygium, *Figure 9.6*) and neoplastic (e.g. ocular surface squamous neoplasia, *Figure 9.7*). A thorough history would give clues to diagnosis, but only through examination can a firm diagnosis be made. Conjunctival lesions may or may not be apparent with the use of a pen torch for a close inspection, and therefore only slit lamp examination can allow the ophthalmologist to look for features indicative of a particular diagnosis.

History

The determination of the need for referral to your local ocular surface service may be determined by asking the following questions:
- Change in size?
- Change in colour?
- Increased redness?
- Pain?
- Changes in vision?
- Is there any sign or symptom of infection or inflammation (photophobia or light sensitivity, eye redness)?

Management

Referrals are made on the basis of:
- Acute symptoms (such as pain, increased redness or drop in vision) which should be made for review on a **same day referral**
- Any concern for malignancy should be referred to **fast-track clinic**
- Asymptomatic pinguecula and pterygia **do not require referral**
  ○ irritative symptoms:

- lubricating eye drops
- **refer routinely** for ophthalmology review to consider topical steroids
  - ○ pterygia can be **routinely referred** for consideration for surgery if causing significant astigmatism or refractory discomfort, or if they are encroaching on the visual axis.

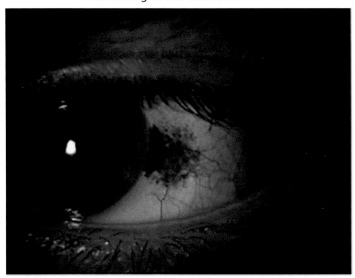

Figure 9.4 Conjunctival naevus; cysts and lack of feeder vessels are a reassuring sign. Usually present from childhood, may increase in size / darken during puberty.

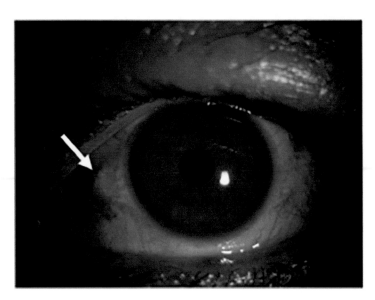

Figure 9.5 Pinguecula of nasal conjunctiva (white arrow).

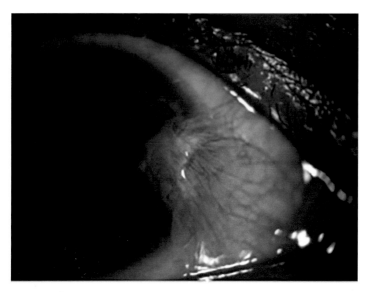

Figure 9.6 Pterygium.

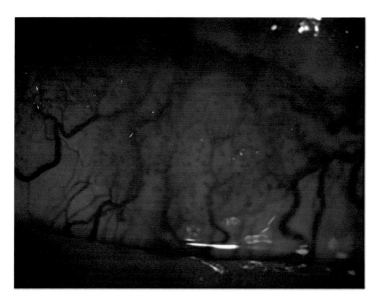

Figure 9.7 Ocular surface squamous neoplasia: conjunctival intraepithelial neoplasia (gelatinous, vascularized mass with feeder vessels. Requires topical chemotherapy / immunotherapy and a 'no-touch' surgical excision.

9.4 Corneal ulcers

Corneal ulcers can have devastating consequences for the sight of a patient. Risk factors include contact lens wear, trauma, ocular surface disease, lid disease, nasolacrimal duct disease, immunosuppression and nutritional deficiency.

History
Ask about:

- Onset and duration
- Pain
- Red eye
- Eyelid swelling, redness or malposition
- Reduced vision
- Discharge
- Photophobia
- Trauma
- Contact lens wear
- Dry eye disease
- Immunosuppression
- Malnutrition.

RED FLAG

All contact lens wearers with a red painful eye must be referred the same day to local eye services.

 All patients suspected of having a corneal ulcer need **immediate referral** to eye services so that the correct treatment can be instigated. *Section 2.4* indicates how assessment of the anterior segment without a slit lamp can be performed.

 ## Examination
Examination should include baseline visual acuity and IOP.

- Assess:
  - type of corneal ulcer (an epithelial defect with underlying stromal infiltrate)
  - depth (does it affect all layers of the cornea?)
  - evidence of thinning
  - Seidel's sign (leak from anterior chamber due to perforated cornea) with fluorescein 2% instilled
  - foreign body
  - anterior chamber activity (cells or flare)
  - hypopyon
- Look for eyelid disease
- Palpate lacrimal sac for regurgitation.

Investigations

- Corneal ulcers >1.5mm in diameter should be scraped for microbiology analysis (see *Box 9.1* for corneal scrape technique).

Management

- Treatment is instigated based on local cornea and microbiology guidelines. Choice of agents for topical antibiotic treatment include fluoroquinolones such as levofloxacin or fortified cephalosporins such as cefuroxime.

CLINICAL CONTEXT TIPS

Patient advice on treatment for corneal ulcer
Warn the patient they may have to treat with drops hourly day and night for the first 48 hours.

- Cycloplegia (e.g. cyclopentolate 1%) should also be included for pain management.
- Criteria for admission include:
  - corneal ulcer >1.5mm with central location and complicated by hypopyon or perforation (impending or frank)
  - patients not able to physically administer the drops independently, or those who do not have a support system at home to help them
  - poor compliance
  - monocular patient
  - limited improvement.

CLINICAL CONTEXT TIPS

Assessment of patient for intensive drop instillation
If there is any doubt about the patient's ability to self-administer drops, test this in the clinical area. Also check that carers assisting patients are able to administer the drops correctly.

- Follow-up is intensive for the first 24–48 hours. If there is improvement then the follow-up period can be extended.

CLINICAL CONTEXT TIPS

Social consideration for patient with corneal ulcer
Assess the patient's transport situation for returning for review in the acute phase. There should be a low threshold for admission if the patient will have issues returning for clinical review.

- Advise the patient of the importance of compliance (*"this condition is potentially blinding if we do not control it now"*).

- Specialist cornea advice should be sought if the clinical presentation is not typical, there is no improvement despite good compliance with treatment, in cases of impending or frank perforation, or concern for *Acanthamoeba* keratitis in a contact lens wearer.

BOX 9.1: CORNEAL SCRAPE TECHNIQUE

 Corneal scrapes should only be performed by an ophthalmologist. Depending on the clinical picture, advice should be sought from your local microbiology department on what should be used to capture the sample.

1. Ensure that the procedure is explained to the patient and consent given.
2. Reiterate the importance of keeping still to the patient to ensure safety during the procedure.
3. Position the patient on the slit lamp.
4. Have a low threshold for using an eyelid speculum to keep eyelids open.
5. Instil preservative-free topical anaesthetic to the eye to be sampled.
6. Example of the equipment required to capture the sample is as follows (**NB**: each eye service will have a standard protocol for sending corneal scrapes to microbiology, so be sure to consult with local guidelines. For fungi and *Acanthamoeba*, confocal microscopy is the non-invasive diagnostic tool of choice):
   o Glass slide for microscopy and staining (circle the area where the sample is on the slide with a permanent marker pen)
   o Blood agar (for most bacteria and fungi, including bacteria demonstrating haemolysis)
   o Chocolate agar (for *Haemophilus, Neisseria* and *Moraxella*)
   o Sabouraud agar (for fungi).
7. Use, for example, a 25G needle (again, consult with your local cornea service to gain advice on the best equipment to use) to collect the sample.
8. Use a new needle for each sample collected.
9. Take the sample from the area of the ulcer with the greatest microbe load, e.g. the base or the edge of the ulcer.
10. Ensure all samples are appropriately labelled before sending the sample to your local microbiology department.
11. Advise the patient to continue with topical medication pending microbiology report.

9.4.1 Aetiology

Corneal ulcers can be bacterial, viral, fungal, inflammatory or due to contact lens related keratitis (*Table 9.2*).

Table 9.2 Key features of corneal ulcers

Aetiology	Key features
Bacterial	Circumcorneal injection Epithelial defect Stromal opacity (white/yellow/grey) Anterior uveitis / hypopyon Aetiology • Gram +ve (*Staph. aureus, Staph. epidermidis, Strep. pneumoniae*) • Gram −ve (*P. aeruginosa, N. gonorrhoeae, Haemophilus*)
Viral	Spectrum • Blepharoconjunctivitis • Epithelial involvement (see image; dendritic lesion or geographic ulcer) • Stromal keratitis (stromal oedema and opacity) • Disciform keratitis (endothelial involvement) Aetiology • Herpes simplex (pictured) • Herpes zoster
Fungal	Insidious or rapid onset Feathery branching or satellite lesions Anterior uveitis / hypopyon

Aetiology	Key features
Contact lens related keratitis 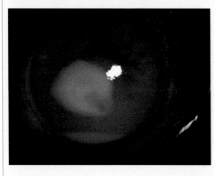	Rapid onset in a contact lens wearer Central location Epithelial defect Corneal thinning Ring-like stromal infiltrate Anterior uveitis / hypopyon Aetiology – often bacterial but can be amoebic ● *P. aeruginosa* (pictured) ● *Acanthamoeba*: insidious onset differentiates it from other aetiologies

---

BOX 9.2: ADVICE TO CONTACT LENS WEARERS

● No swimming, showering or sleeping in lenses (the 3 Ss)
● Do not insert contact lens if eye is red, irritated or painful
● Always have a spare pair of glasses at home for times when contact lens wear is not possible.

9.5 Peripheral corneal disease

Peripheral corneal disease (*Figure 9.8*) occurs where there is peripheral corneal ulceration of varying degrees; this can be in isolation or due to life-threatening systemic conditions.

 Peripheral corneal disease requires in-depth examination by an ophthalmologist at the slit lamp. The role of non-ophthalmic colleagues is to recognize that this condition should not be treated in the community.

9.5.1 Marginal keratitis

● Marginal keratitis occurs as a sequela to lid margin disease (which can occur due to blepharitis, atopy and rosacea) and a hypersensitivity reaction to *Staphylococcus* microbes on the lid – i.e. an inflammation, not a frank infection.
● Patients will present with foreign body sensation, sectoral redness, pain or discomfort.
● The clinical features include a peripheral corneal infiltrate, with overlying epithelial ulceration.
● The key distinguishing feature on slit lamp examination is an area of clear cornea between the area of ulceration and the limbus.
● Treatment is with a combination of topical corticosteroid and antibiotic, but the offending lid disease must also be treated.

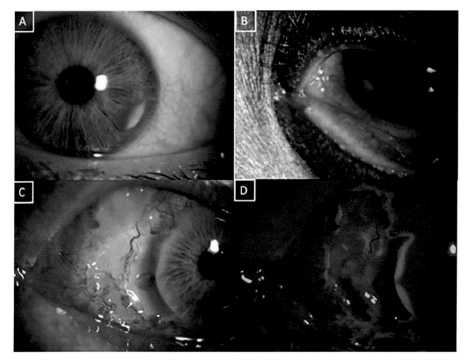

Figure 9.8 Peripheral corneal disease. (A) marginal keratitis; (B) phlyctenulosis; (C) peripheral ulcerative keratitis; (D) peripheral ulcerative keratitis (stained with fluorescein 2% and visualized with blue cobalt light).

- Referral to ophthalmology from non-ophthalmic services should be **within 24 hours if new presentation, or within 48 hours if the patient has a previous history**.

9.5.2 Phlyctenulosis

- Phlyctenulosis is also due to a staphylococcal hypersensitivity response, but is mostly found in children with a history of blepharokeratoconjunctivitis.
- The child may present with a history of pain (although many children will not complain of pain), photophobia and redness of the eye which remains despite treatment with topical antibiotics. These patients require **same day referral** to local eye services to prevent further involvement of the cornea, which can lead to further permanent reduced vision.
- On slit lamp examination, the phlycten can involve the conjunctiva, cornea or both. Corneal involvement normally exhibits grey nodules of the peripheral cornea, with superficial vascularization extending from the limbus to the cornea.
- Treatment involves aggressive lid hygiene and a combination of systemic antibiotics, with topical corticosteroids and artificial tears.

9.5.3 Peripheral ulcerative keratitis

- Peripheral ulcerative keratitis (PUK) is a sight-threatening form of peripheral corneal disease. It is often associated with systemic inflammatory conditions such as rheumatoid arthritis (RA; see *Chapter 21*) and granulomatosis with polyangiitis (GPA, a life-threatening condition; see *Chapter 21*).
- The patient presents with mild to moderate pain and reduced vision.
- Assessment of the area of epithelial and stromal thinning is best done under slit lamp visualization with fluorescein 2% (particularly looking for Seidel's sign).
- PUK must be considered in a patient with a painful red eye with a background of a systemic autoimmune / inflammatory disease.
- **Same day referral** to local emergency eye services.
- Patients need aggressive immunosuppressive treatment, which will often require the assistance of rheumatology colleagues.

9.6 Corneal graft

Corneal graft is a surgical technique used to improve the corneal surface, improving visual function. Diseased cornea is removed and replaced with donor cornea. A corneal graft can be full thickness (penetrating keratoplasty; *Figure 9.9*), lamellar (deep anterior lamellar keratoplasty, superficial anterior lamellar keratoplasty or endothelial keratoplasty, Descemet's stripping endothelial keratoplasty; *Figure 9.10*). If sutures are seen on the cornea, as in *Figure 9.9*, the patient is likely to have undergone either a penetrating keratoplasty or a deep or superficial anterior lamellar keratoplasty.

Patients who have undergone corneal graft are normally required to continue with topical corticosteroid eye drops long-term. Clinicians in primary care and A&E can help reiterate the importance of compliance for these patients, particularly when refills are requested through their GP, and when cornea service visits are only annual

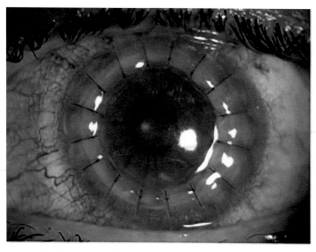

Figure 9.9 Penetrating keratoplasty.

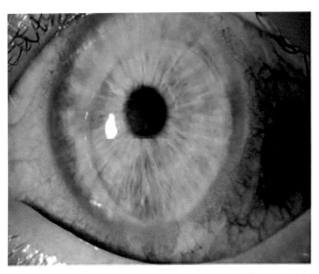

Figure 9.10 Descemet's stripping endothelial keratoplasty (DSEK).

because patients are clinically stable. Any query or concern with the use of long-term corticosteroid eye drops should be directed to the patient's cornea specialist, because stopping the medication puts the patient at risk of corneal rejection (*Figure 9.11*) or failure. *Table 9.3* gives a summary of the type of complications that can occur with corneal graft surgery.

Table 9.3 Corneal graft complications

Early complications	Late complications	Rejection
Wound leak	Suture-related	Immune-mediated response (unlike failure)
Raised IOP	Microbial keratitis	
Primary failure (corneal oedema that never resolves from day 1 post-op, non-immune-mediated)	Late failure	Can be early or late
	Disease recurrence in the graft	Site-dependent
		● Epithelial
Endophthalmitis		● Stromal (subepithelial infiltrates)
Persistent epithelial defect (duration >2 weeks)		● Endothelial (corneal oedema, keratic precipitates, inflammatory demarcation line)

Treatment of suspected graft rejection is with aggressive topical corticosteroids in the first instance. It is imperative to **refer same day** to your local eye service if there is suspicion of this clinical presentation.

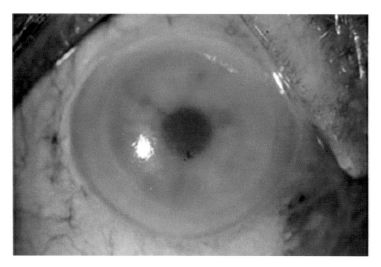

Figure 9.11 Corneal graft rejection in a patient who had a DSEK procedure.

RED FLAG

A patient presenting with a red, painful eye and photophobia on a background of a corneal transplant should be referred to eye services for same day review, due to the risk of infection, rejection or failure. It should never be treated as conjunctivitis in the community.

9.7 Corneal dystrophies

Table 9.4 illustrates the commonest dystrophies (a group of inherited, non-inflammatory, bilateral disorders) that can affect each layer of the cornea.

CLINICAL CONTEXT TIPS

What is recurrent corneal erosion syndrome?
Recurrent corneal erosion is a debilitating disorder caused by spontaneous breakdown of the corneal epithelium, often waking the patient at night. The patient often has a history of sharp trauma previously (think baby accidentally scratching the eye of parent), corneal dystrophies (see Table 9.4) or severe dry eye.

- The mainstay of treatment with acute presentation is aggressive use of artificial tears and cycloplegia
- Bandage contact lens with topical antibiotic cover can also be beneficial and applied in the ophthalmology setting
- Frequent episodes warrant referral to the cornea service for consideration of alcohol delamination of the epithelium.

Table 9.4 Common corneal dystrophies

Dystrophy	Inheritance and onset	Features	Treatment
Epithelium and Bowman's layer			
Epithelial basement membrane dystrophy (map-dot-fingerprint dystrophy) – most common	AD; early adulthood	Bilateral Asymmetrical Faint opacities Microcysts Curvilinear ridges Recurrent corneal erosions	Treat recurrent corneal erosion (see *Clinical Context Tips* below)
Reis–Bücklers	AD; early childhood	Bilateral Central reticular cloudiness of the cornea causing reduced vision Frequent episodes of recurrent corneal erosion	Treat recurrent corneal erosion (see *Clinical Context Tips* below) Laser keratectomy Corneal graft
Meesmann	AD; first year of life	Bilateral Intraepithelial cysts	Mostly asymptomatic
Stroma			
Lattice (most common)	AD	Bilateral Asymmetric Amyloid deposition Type I (commonest) only in the eye Type II familial systemic amyloidosis Type III occurs in patients of Japanese origin Filamentous / criss-cross lesions Recurrent corneal erosions	Treat recurrent corneal erosion (see *Clinical Context Tips* below) Laser keratectomy Corneal graft

Dystrophy	Inheritance and onset	Features	Treatment
Granular	AD	Bilateral Asymmetric White dots and stellate-like opacities with clear surrounding cornea Recurrent corneal erosions	Treat recurrent corneal erosion (see *Clinical Context Tips* below) Corneal graft
Avellino	AD	Bilateral Asymmetric Combination of lattice and granular dystrophy features Recurrent corneal erosions	Treat recurrent corneal erosion (see *Clinical Context Tips* below) Corneal graft
Endothelial			
Fuchs' endothelial dystrophy	AD or sporadic; gradual presentation with increasing age	Worsening vision, particularly in the morning Corneal guttata Stromal oedema Recurrent corneal erosions Stromal haze	5% sodium chloride to reduce oedema Bandage contact lens for comfort Corneal graft Risk of corneal decompensation with cataract surgery so important to counsel patient

AD, autosomal dominant.

9.8 Scleritis

The anatomy of the sclera is discussed in *Section 2.6*. Inflammation of the sclera can result from autoimmune inflammatory conditions or infection. Although scleritis is the inflammation of the tough fibrous coat of the globe (*Figure 9.12*), episcleritis is inflammation of a fibroelastic structure between the conjunctiva and the sclera. The main differences between episcleritis and scleritis in clinical presentation are:
- Pain: patients with scleritis are in immense pain (*"does the eye pain keep you up at night?"*)

- Redness: patients with episcleritis would have a bright red or pink colour to the diffuse or sectoral injection of the eye, whilst patients with scleritis have a darker red colour
- Tenderness: gentle palpation of the globe is not tolerated in patients with scleritis.

Management
See *Chapters 21* and *22*.

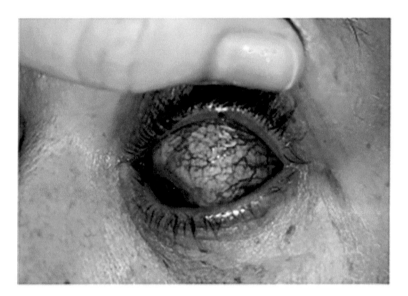

Figure 9.12 Scleritis.

Chapter 10

Anterior chamber and iridocorneal angle

10.1 Introduction

Chapter 2 provided an introduction to the anatomy of the anterior chamber (see *Figure 2.15*) and the iridocorneal angle (see *Figure 2.16*). The anterior chamber is a part of the eye that can be visualized without the use of a slit lamp looking for macroscopic pathology, whilst microscopic pathology requires the use of a slit lamp. This chapter describes uveitis and glaucoma, two of the more common conditions that have clinical findings in the anterior chamber and the iridocorneal angle.

10.2 Uveitis

10.2.1 Introduction

Uveitis is inflammation of the uveal tract (iris, ciliary body and choroid). It can be described as anterior, intermediate (affecting the vitreous), or posterior uveitis (involvement of the choroid and/or the retina), or panuveitis when it affects the whole eye. Uveitis can also be either non-infectious (and associated with systemic disease), infectious or idiopathic. The text below highlights how the primary site of inflammation links to the likely aetiology (see Burkholder and Jabs (2021) for more detail).

- Anterior uveitis
  - primary site of inflammation: anterior chamber
  - non-infectious disease: HLA-B27-associated, juvenile idiopathic arthritis, sarcoidosis, Behçet's disease
  - infectious disease: herpes simplex virus (HSV), varicella zoster virus (VZV), cytomegalovirus, syphilis
  - eye-specific: Fuchs heterochromic iridocyclitis
- Intermediate uveitis
  - primary site of inflammation: vitreous
  - non-infectious disease: multiple sclerosis, sarcoidosis, tubulointerstitial nephritis
  - infectious disease: syphilis, Lyme disease
  - eye-specific: pars planitis
- Posterior uveitis
  - primary site of inflammation: retina and/or choroid
  - non-infectious disease: sarcoidosis
  - infectious disease: toxoplasmosis, tuberculosis, syphilis, cytomegalovirus, acute retinal necrosis (herpes or varicella), *Bartonella*, Lyme disease, fungal (candida, aspergillosis)
  - eye-specific: 'white dot' syndromes

- Panuveitis
  - primary site of inflammation: all of uveal tract, including vitreous and retina
  - non-infectious disease: sarcoid, Behçet's disease, Vogt–Koyanagi–Harada disease
  - infectious disease: syphilis, Lyme disease
  - eye-specific: sympathetic ophthalmia.

 The work-up of a patient with uveitis is performed in an ophthalmology clinic. This includes history, systems review, examination and auxiliary testing. Uveitis can have profound ocular morbidity for patients, and complications such as refractory uveitis (i.e. non-responsive to treatment), glaucoma, permanent sight loss and loss of the eye can occur if uveitis is not treated expeditiously. The role of the non-ophthalmic clinician is to delineate from the information given in the history whether the patient has presented with uveitis and, if so, to make a **same day referral** to ophthalmology.

History

These symptoms are similar to corneal symptoms; however, with corneal pathology, you will see signs (e.g. foreign body, keratitis, ulcer or abrasion) on the cornea.

Ask about:

- Any pain, photophobia or blurred vision accompanying redness of the eye
- Any floaters or blurred vision / loss of vision
- Any recent trauma
- Previous ocular surgery
- Any past medical history of the following:
  - ankylosing spondylitis
  - inflammatory bowel disease
  - juvenile idiopathic arthritis
  - infectious diseases (herpes simplex, varicella zoster, human immunodeficiency virus / acquired immune deficiency syndrome (HIV/AIDS), tuberculosis, syphilis, etc.)
  - psoriasis
  - sarcoidosis
  - malignancy
- Drug history
  - bisphosphonates
  - sulfonamides
  - moxifloxacin
  - over-the-counter / herbal medications
- Social history
  - intravenous drug use.

 For the ophthalmologist, including a systems-based approach with a complete history is useful to rule out (or rule in) the cause of uveitis in a patient. *Box 10.1* provides a guide to questions that are useful for each system.

BOX 10.1: SYSTEMS REVIEW OF THE UVEITIS PATIENT

General health
- Malaise
- Weight loss
- Loss of appetite
- Night sweats
- Enlarged lymph nodes

Cardiovascular system	**Respiratory system**	**GI system**	**Genito-urinary system**
- Chest pain (at rest and/or exertion) - Irregular heartbeat - Pitting oedema of the legs - Evidence of deep vein thrombosis	- Cough (dry/productive) - Blood-stained/green phlegm - Shortness of breath	- Diarrhoea - Nausea and vomiting - Blood/mucus in stool - Jaundice	- Pain on passing urine - Blood or pus in urine - Genital ulcers

Skin	**Musculoskeletal**	**Central nervous system**	**ENT**
- Rashes (vesicular, plaque) - Loss of skin pigment (vitiligo) - Loss of hair (alopecia)	- Joint pain - Joint redness - Lower back pain	- Headache - Seizures - Loss of consciousness - Paraesthesia - Loss of sensation - Bowel and bladder incontinence	- Hearing loss - Mouth ulcers - Recurrent nosebleeds - Sinusitis - Earlobe pain and swelling

Examination

Assess:
- Vision
- Colour vision
- Intraocular pressure
- Fields to confrontation.

Inflammation of the eye leads to disruption of the blood–aqueous barrier, causing an influx of inflammatory cells and protein into the anterior chamber. This leads to clinical findings known as cells and flare (turbidity and haziness of the aqueous humour). Conditions other than uveitis that can lead to the influx of these cells are corneal ulcers (see *Chapter 9*), trauma (see *Chapter 16*) and endophthalmitis (see *Chapter 11*).

Assess for:

- Cells: requires visualization with the slit lamp with a small (1mm × 1mm) beam of light, at a 45° angle and with high magnification; seen as tiny reflective objects floating in the aqueous humour (*Figure 10.1A*)
- Flare
- Keratic precipitates (KPs): aggregate of inflammatory cells sticking to the endothelium (*Figure 10.1B*)
  - smaller KPs = non-granulomatous inflammatory process
  - large KPs ('mutton fat') = granulomatous inflammation
- Hypopyon: aggregation and sedimentation of inflammatory cells (*Figure 10.1C*)
- Hypopyon and red blood cells (*Figure 10.1D*).

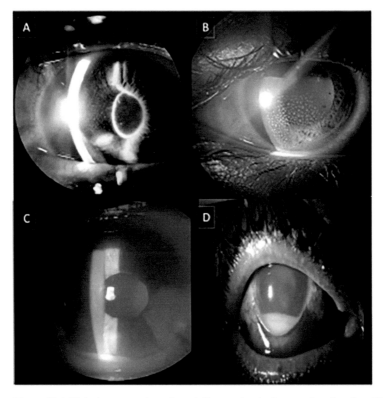

Figure 10.1 Clinical presentation of eye inflammation in the anterior chamber. (A) Anterior chamber cells (white specks between corneal slit lamp beam and lens); (B) keratic precipitates; (C) inferior hypopyon; (D) inferior hypopyon mixed with red blood cells.

CLINICAL CONTEXT TIPS

How to visualize cells in the anterior chamber
Visualization of cells in the anterior chamber requires a slit lamp, except for a hypopyon, which may be recognized using only a pen torch. If the inferior part of the iris is covered with a yellowish–white substance in a red painful eye, think of an ulcer or a hypopyon and refer the patient the **same day** to your emergency eye service.

Ophthalmologists use the Standardization of Uveitis Nomenclature (SUN) criteria to quantify cells and flare in the anterior chamber (grading 0 to 4+ with increasing intensity) and of vitreous haze (grading 0 to 4+ with increasing intensity). *Table 10.1* describes the differences between the classifications.

RED FLAG

A child with a recent diagnosis of juvenile idiopathic arthritis requires review by an ophthalmologist to be screened for uveitis within 6 weeks of referral. This is because children with uveitis and juvenile idiopathic arthritis are often asymptomatic. If a child presents with an abnormal red reflex (due to band keratopathy, synechiae or cataract) in this setting, then they should be reviewed by an ophthalmologist within one week of referral.

Table 10.1 Quantification and grading of clinical features in a patient with uveitis

Cells		Flare		Vitreous haze	
Grade	Description (cells in the field)	Grade	Description	Grade	Description
0	<1	0	None	0	None
0.5+	1–5			0.5+	Slight blurring of optic disc margins
1+	6–15	1+	Faint	1+	Mild blurring of optic disc and retinal vessels
2+	16–25	2+	Moderate (iris and lens clear)	2+	Marked blurring of optic disc and retinal vessels
3+	26–50	3+	Marked (iris and lens hazy)	3+	Optic disc visible but no retinal vessel visible (think light from lighthouse in dense fog)
4+	>50	4+	Intense (difficult to visualize iris details)	4+	Optic disc not visible

Adapted from data in Jabs *et al.* (2005) with permission from Elsevier.

Other important anterior segment findings related to uveitis are:
- Synechiae (where the iris is stuck to the anterior capsule of the lens and may appear poorly reactive or small)
- Iris nodules (Koeppe or Busacca)
- Iris atrophy (common in HSV and VZV unilateral uveitis).

On dilated fundus examination look for:
- Optic disc swelling
- Indistinct or white edges to the retinal vessels (*think vasculitis*)
- Indistinct white or yellow lesions of the retina or choroid (*think retinitis or choroiditis*).

CLINICAL CONTEXT TIPS

When to consider a uveitis with a viral aetiology
In patients presenting with anterior uveitis and raised intraocular pressure, consider a viral aetiology.

Investigation

Investigation of uveitis is particularly selective. The anatomical location, clinical features and laterality of uveitis can determine what investigations are performed to aid diagnosis and management. Infectious causes of uveitis require antimicrobial treatment, and so serology tests are key to ensuring the right treatment for the right aetiology. It is also important to recognize that masquerade conditions such as lymphoma can also cause uveitis. *Chapters 21* and *22* discuss the clinical findings for infectious and non-infectious causes of uveitis. *Table 10.2* provides an A–Z guide to laboratory tests depending on the suspected aetiology of the uveitis.

Table 10.2 A–Z of investigations required for infectious and non-infectious uveitis

Suspected aetiology	Investigations
Birdshot chorioretinopathy	Electrophysiology
	HLA-A29
Demyelination (multiple sclerosis)	MRI looking for hyperintense periventricular white matter lesions
	Lumbar puncture (looking for oligoclonal bands)
Juvenile idiopathic arthritis	Antinuclear antibodies (ANA)
Lyme disease	*Borrelia* serology
Lymphoma	Vitreous biopsy
	MRI head scan

Suspected aetiology	Investigations
Sarcoidosis	Angiotensin-converting enzyme (ACE)
	Chest X-ray
	High resolution CT scan of chest
	MRI head (when suspecting neurosarcoid)
Syphilis	**Step 1: non-treponemal blood test** Venereal disease research laboratory (VDRL) Rapid plasma reagin (RPR) If positive, confirm with: **Step 2: treponemal blood test** Fluorescent treponemal antibody test absorption (FTA-ABS)
Tubulointerstitial nephritis and uveitis syndrome (TINU)	Beta-2 microglobulin
Toxocariasis	*Toxocara* enzyme-linked immunoassay
Toxoplasmosis	*Toxoplasma* IgM and IgG
Tuberculosis	Chest X-ray
	Tuberculin skin test
	Interferon-gamma release assays (IGRAs)
Viral (herpes simplex, varicella zoster, cytomegalovirus)	Viral PCR on diagnostic paracentesis (aqueous humour tap)

Management

Treatment is guided by the clinical suspicion of the underlying aetiology. Treatment should only be instigated by an ophthalmologist, and the expertise of a uveitis specialist should be sought when there is lack of clarity as to the aetiology and/ or poor treatment response. Medical treatment is normally in the form of frequent topical corticosteroids, e.g. dexamethasone or prednisolone 1% starting at 1–2 hourly with a taper, with cycloplegia (cyclopentolate 1% 3×/day or atropine 1% 2×/day) to break or prevent synechiae. With infectious uveitis, systemic antimicrobials need to be considered in combination with topical or systemic corticosteroid treatment, and intravitreal corticosteroids also have a role in non-infectious posterior uveitis.

Complications

- Cataract
- Cystoid macular oedema
- Uveitic glaucoma
- Choroidal neovascularization
- Retinal scars.

10.3 Glaucoma

10.3.1 Introduction

Glaucoma is a progressive optic neuropathy (damage to the optic nerve) with visual field defects (see *Chapter 17*), and with increased intraocular pressure (IOP) being a risk factor. Many people presume raised IOP and glaucoma are synonymous, but they are not. Glaucoma can only be diagnosed when there is evidence of optic nerve damage over time. If IOP is high without damage to the optic nerve, this is ocular hypertension (OHT). If IOP is within normal range with glaucomatous changes to the disc, this is normal-tension glaucoma (see *Table 10.3*).

Glaucoma can be due to a primary or secondary aetiology. *Table 10.3* describes the different classifications of glaucoma and their key clinical features. The work-up of glaucoma patients occurs with eye specialists, but in primary care and A&E it is important to recognize those patients at risk of glaucoma (strong family history, high far-sightedness, high near-sightedness, trauma). It is even more important to recognize patients who may be having acute episodes of increased intraocular pressure / acute angle closure (headaches, haloes around lights, blurred vision, nausea, fixed pupil, often in an older, phakic patient; see *Red flag* box below) which require **immediate referral** to local eye emergency services. Patients with suspected non-acute glaucoma are **referred routinely** to their local eye service.

History

Ask about:
- Any visual symptoms:
  - haloes around lights at night
  - eye pain or headache (particularly at night)
  - subjective visual field loss
- Ocular history:
  - refractive error
  - retinal vascular occlusion
  - surgery
  - trauma
  - uveitis
- Past medical history:
  - COPD / asthma (very important before prescribing beta-blockers)
  - ischaemic heart disease
  - obstructive sleep apnoea
  - stroke
- Family history of glaucoma:
  - age of onset
  - blindness from glaucoma
- Medication history, drug use – particularly steroids or those that can cause acute angle closure:
  - antihistamines such as promethazine
  - topiramate
  - tricyclic antidepressants.

Table 10.3 Classifications of glaucoma and key clinical features

Classification	Sub-category	Clinical features
Ocular hypertension (OHT)		IOP >24mmHg No optic disc cupping No changes on visual fields
Open angle		
Primary	Primary open angle glaucoma (POAG)	No underlying ocular condition IOP >24mmHg
	Normal tension glaucoma (NTG)	No underlying ocular condition IOP <24mmHg
Secondary	Pseudoexfoliation (PXF)	Age >40 years Female Fibrillar deposits in anterior segment of eye Heavily pigmented trabecular meshwork Also, fibrillar deposits in the cardiovascular and cerebrovascular systems (increased risk of heart attack and stroke)
	Pigment dispersion	Age <40 years Male Myopia Pigment on corneal endothelium ('Krukenberg spindle') Heavily pigmented trabecular meshwork Mid-periphery spoke-like iris transillumination
	Inflammatory	Any age Elevated IOP (>35mmHg) Evidence of inflammation in the AC (cells and flare) Posner–Schlossman (high IOP of 40–50mmHg, minimal inflammation in the AC) Fuchs heterochromic uveitis (raised IOP (>35mmHg), minimal injection, stellate KPs, iris atrophy and heterochromia, cataract)

Table 10.3 *cont'd*

Classification	Sub-category	Clinical features
Secondary *cont'd*	Steroid-induced	Any age Topical (or occasionally systemic) corticosteroid use (can occur as soon as 4 days after starting the drops)
	Lens-related	Age >50 years Phacolytic: hypermature cataract Release of lens proteins into the AC, which blocks the trabecular meshwork
	Red cell	Any age Hyphaema (micro- or macro-) Blocks trabecular meshwork
	Angle recession	Any age Blunt trauma related Tear between iris root and ciliary body on gonioscopy
Closed angle		
Primary	Primary angle closure	Age >40 years Hypermetropes Narrow or closed angle on gonioscopy
Secondary	Inflammatory	Any age Increased IOP Shallow AC due to angle closure from iris bombe or synechiae in the angle
	Neovascular	Age >50 years Retinal vascular occlusion (particularly central retinal vein occlusion; see *Chapter 12*) Elevated IOP (>40mmHg) Pain New vessels in the iridocorneal angle on gonioscopy
	Lens-related	Age >50 years Phacomorphic: large cataractous lens Elevated IOP Shallow AC Opposite eye has a deep AC (see Red flag box on acute angle closure below)

Examination

An examination for patients suspected of having glaucoma needs to take place in an eye service setting. Non-ophthalmic clinicians should recognize the signs and symptoms of acute angle closure (see *Red flag* box below), and patients at high risk of glaucoma.

Assess:
- Visual acuity
- Colour vision
- Intraocular pressure (with Goldmann tonometry)
- Central corneal thickness (as this can cause over- or under-estimation of the IOP)
- Gonioscopy to identify features of the iridocorneal angle that are contributing to the underlying pathology (*Figure 10.2* illustrates the difference between an open angle and a closed angle)
- Pupillary responses (including any relative afferent pupillary defect)
- Visual fields (which should be by formal perimetry; see *Chapter 17*)
- Optical coherence tomography (OCT) if available (see *Chapter 18*)
- Dilated fundus examination: assessment of the optic disc, looking for cupping of the optic disc, as well as other signs of glaucomatous changes (namely notching of the neuroretinal rim which indicates loss of cells, and baring and bayoneting of the optic disc vessels and nasal displacement (nasalization) of the optic disc vessels; see *Figure 10.3*).

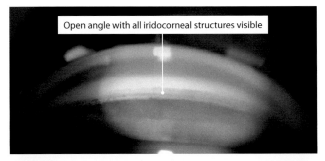

Open angle with all iridocorneal structures visible

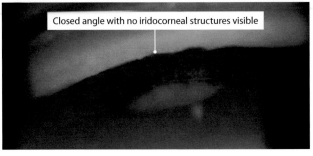

Closed angle with no iridocorneal structures visible

Figure 10.2 Gonioscopy findings in open and closed angle.

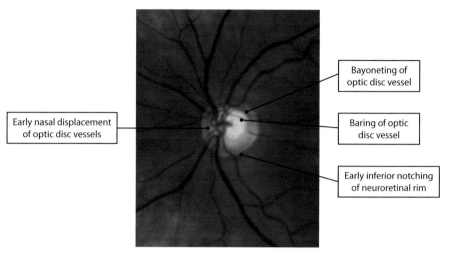

Bayoneting of optic disc vessel

Early nasal displacement of optic disc vessels

Baring of optic disc vessel

Early inferior notching of neuroretinal rim

Figure 10.3 Glaucomatous optic disc.

RED FLAG

Acute intraocular pressure rise, particularly acute angle closure, is an ophthalmic emergency.

History:
- Red painful eye
- Headache
- Haloes around lights
- Loss of vision
- Nausea and vomiting.

Examination:
- Red eye
- Hazy cornea (*is there asymmetry to how well the iris details can be seen compared with the other eye?*)
- Fixed dilated pupil.

Immediate referral to the local eye emergency service

Assessment:
- Check **visual acuity**
- Check **IOP** (preferably with Goldmann applanation tonometry)
- Assess the **anterior chamber** and **perform gonioscopy**
  - is the AC shallow?
  - are there cells or flare?
  - is there neovascularization of the iris?
  - is the pupil reactive?

  - o is there neovascularization of the angle on gonioscopy?
  - o is there a large cataractous lens?
- Assess the **contralateral eye**.

Immediate:
- **Stat IV acetazolamide 500mg**
  - o check for history of kidney disease and allergy to sulfa medications
  - o warn patient about frequent urination (especially older men with benign prostatic hypertrophy)
- **Stat topical beta-blocker (timolol 0.5%)**
- **Stat alpha-2 agonist (apraclonidine 1%)**
- **Stat pilocarpine 2% once IOP <40mmHg (only** in primary acute angle closure glaucoma and phacomorphic glaucoma)
  OR
- **Stat cycloplegia** (cyclopentolate 1% or atropine 1%) in acute inflammatory or neovascular glaucoma
- Recheck IOP in 1 hour
- Consider IV mannitol 20% 1–1.5g/kg, if IOP fails to improve
  - o contraindicated in patients with severe renal disease.

Maintenance:
- Oral acetazolamide 250mg
- Maximum topical medication
- Beta-blocker (timolol 0.5%)
- Alpha-2 agonist (apraclonidine 1%)
- Prostaglandin analogues (latanoprost)
- Pilocarpine 2% to **both** eyes in acute primary angle closure.

Definitive treatment:
- Primary angle closure: peripheral iridotomy (consider doing this in the emergency setting if the cornea is clear) or remove cataract if present
- Phacomorphic glaucoma: cataract surgery
- Inflammatory glaucoma: topical corticosteroids and medical anti-glaucoma management
- Neovascular glaucoma: PRP and anti-VEGF to reduce the neovascular drive; medical anti-glaucoma management, topical corticosteroids and cycloplegia; surgical anti-glaucoma management if IOP fails to improve.

CLINICAL CONTEXT TIPS

How to measure intraocular pressure
The gold standard for measuring the intraocular pressure is using Goldmann applanation tonometry, although there are portable contact instruments available that allow quick and easy measurements, e.g. Tonopen and iCare.

Medical management

First-line for OHT and mild to moderate glaucoma are topical anti-glaucoma medications which aim to decrease aqueous production (such as with beta-blockers) or increase aqueous humour outflow (such as with prostaglandin analogues), or both (alpha-2 adrenergic receptor agonist). Patients will often be started on one eye drop (normally a prostaglandin analogue such as latanoprost), and treatment escalates depending on the IOP response. Medications can also be modified depending on how well the patient tolerates them (e.g. shortness of breath with beta-blockers or allergic conjunctivitis with brimonidine).

CLINICAL CONTEXT TIPS

When not to use topical beta-blockers in glaucoma
Topical beta-blockers should be avoided in patients with COPD, asthma, bradycardia, congestive heart failure and heart block, as they can lead to exacerbation or worsening of the medical condition.

Laser management

In OHT and open angle glaucoma, use of a YAG laser (specifically selective laser trabeculoplasty) to the trabecular meshwork causes remodelling, increased aqueous humour outflow and reduced intraocular pressure.

In closed angle glaucoma, a YAG laser is applied to a thin part of the peripheral iris to produce a hole that serves as an alternative pathway for flow of aqueous humour from the anterior to the posterior segment (peripheral iridotomy).

Cyclophotocoagulation (also known as cyclodiode) is generally reserved for patients with uncontrolled intraocular pressure in eyes with poor visual potential. It uses a diode laser to destroy the ciliary body and reduce aqueous humour secretion.

Surgical management

Surgical treatment for glaucoma is often instigated when there is advanced glaucoma, failure of maximum tolerated medical treatment or when patients are unable to take their medications (frail or poor mobility).

Filtration surgery for glaucoma uses an alternative pathway by which aqueous humour can drain and decrease IOP. In trabeculectomy, a partial thickness scleral flap is created to produce a pathway between the anterior chamber and the subconjunctival space for aqueous humour to flow. At the site of the flap, there is an adjacent bleb, which is an elevated area of conjunctiva and signifies the filtration point of aqueous humour. The use of antimetabolites such a 5-fluorouracil and mitomycin C (in so-called augmented trabeculectomy) is to prevent scarring and improve the longevity of the bleb.

Glaucoma drainage implants are prostheses that also provide an alternative aqueous humour drainage pathway. Simplistically, the implant has a silicone tube that is, in

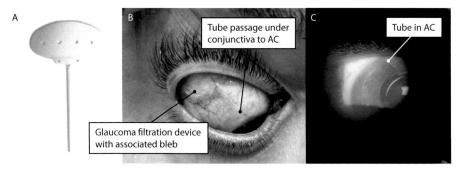

A

B Tube passage under conjunctiva to AC

C Tube in AC

Glaucoma filtration device with associated bleb

Figure 10.4 Glaucoma drainage implant. (A) glaucoma drainage device with end plate and silicone tube; (B) glaucoma drainage device *in situ*; (C) silicone tube in the anterior chamber.

most cases, inserted into the anterior chamber (although it can also be placed in the ciliary sulcus or vitreous cavity), whilst its end-plate is placed in a quadrant (normally the superotemporal quadrant) where it gains a fibrous capsule where aqueous humour pools and passively diffuses from the subconjunctival space into the episcleral venous system (*Figure 10.4*). In recent times, microinvasive glaucoma surgery utilizes small drainage devices that can connect the anterior chamber with Schlemm's canal and improve IOP. These devices can be implanted at the time of cataract surgery.

Table 10.4 illustrates the complications that can arise from laser and surgical treatments for glaucoma.

RED FLAG

Any patient presenting with a red painful eye after laser or surgery for glaucoma should have **immediate referral** to the local ophthalmology department. This is to assess for increased or decreased IOP, as well as blebitis (isolated infection of the bleb) or endophthalmitis.

Table 10.4 Summary of the complications of laser and filtration surgery for glaucoma

Laser	Filtration surgery
Peripheral iridotomy	Early complications
• Bleeding	• Shallow AC
• Inflammation	• Hypotony
• IOP spike	• Wound leak
• Corneal burns	• IOP spike
	• Infection
	• Blebitis: red eye with white bleb **but** treat like endophthalmitis (see *Section 11.5*)
	• Endophthalmitis
	• Vision loss

Table 10.4 *cont'd*

Laser	Filtration surgery
Laser trabeculoplasty • Bleeding • Inflammation • IOP spike	**Late complications** • Bleb failure • Leaky bleb • Blebitis or endophthalmitis (*can occur years after surgery*) • Vision loss
Cyclophotocoagulation • Cataract • Haemorrhage • Hypotony (IOP <6mmHg) • Inflammation • Phthisis (shrunken non-functioning eye) • Sympathetic ophthalmia (severe inflammation in the treated and non-treated eye)	

References and further reading

Alwitry, A. and Kinq, A.J. (2012) Surveillance of late onset bleb leak, blebitis and bleb related endophthalmitis – a UK incidence study. *Graefes Arch Clin Exp Ophthalmol*, **250:** 1231.

British Society of Paediatric and Adolescent Rheumatology (BSPAR) and Royal College of Ophthalmologists (2006) *Guidelines for Screening for Uveitis in Juvenile Idiopathic Arthritis (JIA).* Available at: www.rcophth.ac.uk/wp-content/uploads/2022/02/2006_PROF_046_JuvenileArthritis-updated-crest-2.pdf

Burkholder, B.M. and Jabs, D.A. (2021) Uveitis for the non-ophthalmologist. *BMJ*, **372:** m4979.

Jabs, D.A., Nussenblatt, R.B., Rosenbaum, J.B. *et al.* (2005) Standardization of Uveitis Nomenclature (SUN) for reporting clinical data. *Am J Ophthalmol,* **140:** 509.

NICE (2017, updated 2022) NG81: *Glaucoma: diagnosis and management.*

Vaziri, K., Kishor, K., Schwartz, S.G. *et al.* (2015) Incidence of bleb-associated endophthalmitis in the United States. *Clin Ophthalmol*, **9:** 317.

Chapter 11
Lens

11.1 Introduction

The leading causes of vision impairment worldwide are uncorrected refractive error and cataract. Cataract is the opacification or 'clouding' of the usually clear crystalline lens which is often age-related. Lens anatomy has been covered in *Section 2.9*, and the lens pathology that you are most likely to come across is cataract. Most cataracts are age-related, but congenital, trauma, medical history (e.g. diabetes) and medications all play a role in the formation of cataracts.

The main considerations when assessing and referring patients with cataract is to ensure there is no other significant cause for the patient's symptoms, and that the patient is symptomatic enough to undergo assessment for cataract surgery (surgery which itself is not without risk).

It is important to ensure that:
- The main cause of the patient's symptoms is a cataract
- The patient's visual acuity meets the local/regional protocols for cataract surgery (often 6/12)
- The patient is symptomatic enough and activities of daily living are sufficiently affected to warrant undergoing the risks (see below) of cataract surgery.

Often patients are told by their optician that they have a cataract and presume that it needs to be operated on, which is not always the case. Cataract surgery is also so common, and a day-case operation with a high success rate, that it is often thought of as a 'minor' procedure rather than potentially vision-threatening surgery. It is vital that a patient's work-up from referral to pre-operative consent addresses this.

This chapter focuses on how to work a patient up with age-related cataract.

11.2 Cataract

Figure 11.1 shows the progression of a cataract over time.

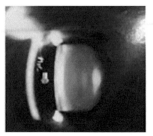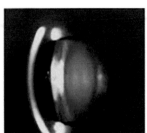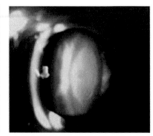

Figure 11.1 Slit lamp photograph showing the progression of a nuclear sclerotic cataract over time.

History

Ask about:
- Gradual, painless reduction of vision
- Glare, particularly when driving at night
- Effect on activities of daily living
- Visual needs for occupation and hobbies.

Ask about:
- Glare (*think cortical and posterior subcapsular cataracts*)
- Reduced contrast sensitivity
- Reduced colour appreciation
- Monocular diplopia
- Ghosting
- Changing astigmatism
- Rule out other causes of gradual vision loss, e.g. scotoma / metamorphopsia (pointing towards macular pathology such as dry age-related macular degeneration).

CLINICAL CONTEXT TIPS

How different symptoms point to different forms of cataract
Nuclear sclerotic cataracts particularly affect distance vision due to the myopic shift. Posterior subcapsular cataracts may be more symptomatic in miosis or bright light. Cortical cataracts are more likely to produce glare, particularly at night.

Broader history is particularly important when considering patients for surgery, in particular:
- Risk factors for cataract:
  - age; if particularly young (i.e. under 40 – although cataracts don't tend to affect vision until age 60 and over)
  - corticosteroid use
  - diabetes
  - known ocular / medical conditions
  - prior trauma
- Risk factors for surgery:
  - patient cooperation (do they have dementia or intellectual disability limiting whether they can follow commands?)
  - hearing
  - positioning ability (are they able to lie flat and still for 30 minutes?)
  - severe COPD (limiting lying flat)
  - medications (specifically alpha-blocker use which can be a risk factor for intraoperative floppy iris syndrome)
  - past medical history of diabetes, hypertension, COPD, history of stroke or myocardial infarction (MI) (general approach is to wait 3–6 months after an MI/ stroke prior to undergoing cataract surgery)

- Risk factors for a guarded prognosis for cataract surgery:
  - current treatment for ocular conditions
  - previous diagnosis of amblyopia
  - previous refractive surgery
  - health of contralateral eye
- Factors affecting post-operative care:
  - is the patient able to instil their own drops?
  - do they have function-limiting arthritis in their hand joints?
  - do they live with someone able to help?

Examination

- Visual acuity
- Pupillary responses
- Note patient's refraction (i.e. glasses prescription)
- Cornea (corneal scarring can be another cause of painless long-standing vision reduction).

- Visual acuity (with and without current glasses and pinhole)
- Refraction
- IOP
- Pupillary responses
- Deep-set orbit
- Eyelid status
  - malposition
  - blepharitis (must be treated prior to cataract surgery to limit infection risk)
- Cornea status
  - scarring
  - guttata (consistent with Fuchs' endothelial dystrophy and which predisposes to corneal decompensation after cataract surgery)
- Anterior chamber depth
- Iatrogenic pupil dilation (is the pupil well dilated or will you need assistance for pupil dilation intraoperatively?)
- Iris
  - iridodonesis (hypermobility of iris)
  - synechiae (iris adhesions to cornea or lens)
  - transillumination (indicating conditions with zonular weakness such as pseudoexfoliation)
- Cataract
- Retinal and optic nerve status (to guide prognosis of cataract surgery).

Investigations

These often take place in a pre-operative assessment cataract clinic and include:
- Refraction
- Biometry (ocular measurements to guide intraocular lens implant choice)
- Optical coherence tomography (OCT) to assess macula and optic disc when necessary).

Management
- Observation if cataract not limiting visual function or if risks outweigh benefit of surgery
- Cataract surgery with implantation of intraocular lens (IOL).

CLINICAL CONTEXT TIPS

How to consent a patient for cataract surgery
Overview to give the patient:

More than 95% of patients have improved eyesight following cataract surgery providing there are no other problems with the eye. In some cases, the vision in the eye may also be poor for other reasons and cataract surgery may not fully improve the vision. There is a very small risk of permanent vision loss (less than 1 in 1000).

Specific risks:
- *1 in 10 patients require a clinic laser treatment at some time in the future to correct 'clouding' of the capsule that the new lens is inserted into. This is generally a well-tolerated, painless 'one-stop' procedure (YAG capsulotomy for posterior capsular opacification).*
- *1 in 20 patients are at risk of complications, which may require further treatment, such as high pressure or inflammation in the eye. These can generally be treated with drops after the procedure.*
- *There is a 1 in 100 risk of requiring an additional procedure at the time of surgery to rectify issues such as a compromise to the delicate structures inside the eye, e.g. the lens capsule (posterior capsule rupture).*
- *There is a 1 in 1000 risk of severe and permanent visual loss due to severe bleeding or infection (suprachoroidal haemorrhage or endophthalmitis).*

Setting patient expectations:

"The artificial lens that we put in place of your cataract can be set to have better focus for either distance (the option most patients choose – which means you will need glasses for reading) or near (a few patients choose this if they perform a lot of detailed close-up work or prefer to read without glasses – in which case you will need glasses for distance). You may also need glasses to correct the vision in general or any astigmatism (a variation in shape of the front of your eye). There is a small chance of needing further corrective surgery if the 'focus outcome' of the new lens is not as expected."

11.3 Pre-operative checks for the ophthalmologist

Same day pre-operative checks for cataract surgery should include:
- Positive patient identification
- Positive procedure confirmation with the patient
- Confirming allergy status (is the patient allergic to latex or shellfish?)
- Ensuring written informed consent has been given

- Marking the side of the procedure
- Ensuring the eye is well dilated
- Checking the eye on the slit lamp to confirm findings and ensure no new ophthalmic problems or lid infections have arisen
- If planned for local anaesthesia, confirming the type of anaesthesia to be used
  - most patients tolerate topical anaesthesia but a subset of patients may require sub-Tenon anaesthetic
  - patients who are particularly sensitive or are likely to attempt to squeeze their eyes shut during the surgery may be better candidates for sub-Tenon anaesthetic
- Confirming that the biometry is accurate and selecting the appropriate intraocular lens implant
- Ensuring the theatre team are aware of the visual acuity in both eyes, the refractive status of both eyes, the intended refractive aim, the intended intraocular lens implant and any patient-specific variations to procedure anticipated, e.g.:
  - intracameral phenylephrine or iris expansion devices for poor dilators
  - intracameral dyes for visualization of the anterior capsule in dense cataracts
  - different types of viscoelastic, e.g. cohesive viscoelastic, to maintain anatomical space within an eye with a smaller anterior chamber depth
- Ensuring the nursing and theatre team are aware of the patient's general medical status and transferring ability (i.e. able to transfer onto the operating table).

Further nursing checks also take place to ensure the patient is systemically well and ready for surgery, in addition to checking that they will be well supported post-operatively.

11.4 Post-operative checks for the ophthalmologist

For uncomplicated cataract surgery, patients often have a 4-week post-operative check at their opticians. Examination should include:
- Visual acuity (unaided + pinhole)
- Refraction
- IOP (watch out for steroid response)
- Corneal clarity and ensuring wounds are clear
- Anterior chamber status (should be deep and relatively quiet)
- Pupil should be round with no vitreous wick to the wound
- Intraocular lens implant well-centred in the lens capsule
- Retina should be flat with a normal foveal contour.

11.5 Post-operative endophthalmitis

Red eye following cataract surgery can be for a variety of reasons including:
- Drop toxicity or allergy to preservatives in drops (often presenting as an itch, irritation or grittiness)
- Post-operative inflammatory reaction (i.e. uveitis) due to reducing or stopping steroid drops (often presenting as a red / sore / photosensitive eye on reduction of drops)

- Raised intraocular pressure (due to retained viscoelastic if the raised IOP presents hours after surgery, or due to steroid response if it presents days to weeks after surgery)
- Retained lens matter.

Endophthalmitis should always be considered for any post-operative (or post-intravitreal injection) patient with a red eye. This is an ophthalmic emergency and should be thought of as the eye version of 'sepsis'. It usually presents within the first week of surgery, so an **emergency referral** for same day review by an ophthalmologist should be made. Note, there are some procedures (e.g. trabeculectomy for glaucoma) where endophthalmitis can present months later, so caution should be exercised in these patients if they present with a red, painful eye.

History

Ask about:
- Pain
- Eyelid swelling
- Red eye
- Loss of vision
- Previous ocular surgery.

Ask about:
- Patient risk factors (blepharitis, pre-operative conjunctivitis, immunocompromised, compliance with drops)
- Surgical risk factors (such as complicated or long surgery).

Examination

- Ensure patient is systemically well
- Note any lid swelling, discharge, visual acuity, pupil assessment.

- Visual acuity (no perception of light has a poorer prognosis)
- IOP
- Conjunctival redness
- Cornea clarity (is the cornea hazy?)
- Cells, flare and hypopyon
- IOL position
- Dilated fundus exam
  - posterior segment inflammation (if no fundal view, use ocular ultrasound (see *Chapter 19*) to assess for vitreous activity and retinal detachment).

Management

Immediate referral to ophthalmology for vitreous sampling and injection of intravitreal antibiotics. Follow local hospital policy to carry out this procedure, but a guide is as follows:
- Call on-call microbiology to ensure they are ready to receive samples
- Call on-call pharmacist to obtain the intravitreal antibiotics

- Perform intravitreal sampling in a clean room (some hospitals advocate for a vitrector biopsy of vitreous in theatres), but not the same room where routine intravitreal injections are performed
- Scrub using sterile gloves and a mask, instil local anaesthetic, prepare (with povidone-iodine) and drape the patient
- Insert eyelid speculum
- Using a 23–25-gauge needle on an insulin syringe, insert 3.5–4mm behind the limbus, aiming into the middle of the vitreous cavity and aspirate 0.2ml of vitreous and send to microbiology for analysis
- Using a separate 27–30-gauge needle, inject intravitreal antibiotics (as per local policy)
- Topical medications include:
  - ○ antibiotics as per local protocol
  - ○ cycloplegia for comfort
- Steroids (topical, intravitreal or systemic) may be used in conjunction with hospital policy and according to clinical picture (e.g. once fungal infection has been excluded and there is improvement at 24 hours)
- Analgesia should be encouraged
- Oral antibiotics are also used as per local hospital policy
- Close monitoring is required with daily review and repeat vitreous sampling + intravitreal antibiotics at 48 hours if there is failure to respond
- Certain patients (e.g. severe vision loss at presentation or failure to respond to repeat intravitreal antibiotics) may be considered for therapeutic vitrectomy
- Cases should be recorded for audit purposes.

11.6 Post-operative considerations for the non-ophthalmologist

Other common post-operative complaints include:
- Floaters: not uncommon after cataract surgery. If there is a sudden shower of floaters, photopsia or shadow / curtain effect **referral to ophthalmology to be seen within 24 hours** is indicated.
- Loss of vision: this has a spectrum of causes (retinal detachment, endophthalmitis, corneal oedema, refractive surprise where the refraction is not as intended) but requires **immediate referral** and same day review by an ophthalmologist.

References and further reading

Endophthalmitis Vitrectomy Study Group (1995) Results of the Endophthalmitis Vitrectomy Study. A randomized trial of immediate vitrectomy and of intravenous antibiotics for the treatment of postoperative bacterial endophthalmitis. *Arch Ophthalmol*, **113**: 1479.

World Health Organization (2021) *Blindness and Vision Impairment*. Available from: www.who.int/news-room/fact-sheets/detail/blindness-and-visual-impairment

Chapter 12
Medical retina

12.1 Introduction

 Many conditions affect the retina, but examination of the retina is difficult for those who either do not have access to, or know how to use, a slit lamp. The most satisfactory way to assess the retina is with dilated fundoscopy, but this option is typically not available in primary care and emergency department settings. As a general rule, medical retina conditions, and in particular macular pathology, cause symptoms of scotoma (central blurring) and metamorphopsia (distortion), but they can also have loss of vision. If the patient has been reviewed by an eye care specialist such as an optician, and a diagnosis confirmed, then the patient can be referred depending on their diagnosis (see *Chapter 6*). However, if the patient is presenting to the GP or A&E with these symptoms, the case should be discussed the **same day** with your local eye department, to determine when the patient should be reviewed.

This chapter discusses the most common medical retina complaints seen in ophthalmology, such as age-related macular degeneration, diabetic retinopathy and vascular occlusions. It will also include a brief overview of inherited retinal dystrophies and ocular oncology.

12.2 Age-related macular degeneration

Age-related macular degeneration (AMD) is the leading cause of irreversible sight loss in those aged over 60. It is an age-related 'wear and tear' of the macula that affects the central vision in the majority of cases. Changes in the physiological balance of the Bruch's membrane / choroid complex cause the deposition of drusen (yellow accumulations of extracellular material between Bruch's membrane and the RPE; see *Section 2.10*) in dry AMD, and choroidal neovascular membrane formation in wet AMD.

NICE (2018) grades AMD as:
- Early AMD
- Late AMD (indeterminate)
- Late AMD (wet active)
- Late AMD (dry)
- Late AMD (wet inactive).

Any one of these diagnoses may have been made by a patient's regular optician. *Figure 12.1* illustrates some AMD subtypes**.** All but asymptomatic early AMD require referral to a hospital eye service for further diagnostic work-up. For patients with a diagnosis of late AMD (wet active), the **referral to your local AMD service should be made within one day of the patient being assessed and diagnosed in primary care, to be seen by ophthalmology within 2 weeks**.

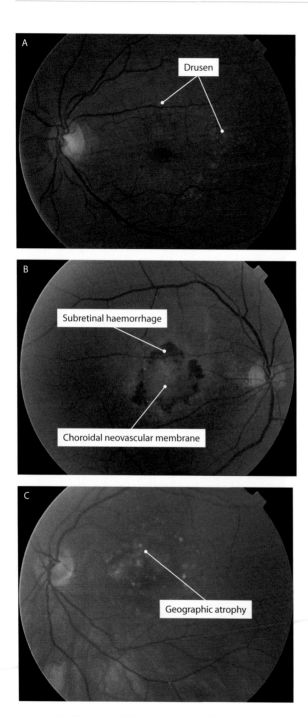

Figure 12.1 Types of AMD: (A) early AMD; (B) late AMD (wet active); (C) late AMD (dry). Images reproduced from www.intechopen.com/chapters/43469 under a CCA BY 3.0 licence.

History

Patients can often present with visual disturbance known as metamorphopsia, where objects appear wavy or distorted. An easy way to assess in any clinical area is by asking the patient to cover one eye and to look at an object with a straight edge such as a door frame. The patient will report that in the centre of their vision, the door frame either appears wavy or a part is missing. If available, an Amsler chart (*Figure 12.2*) is a more formal way of assessing this visual distortion. Other visual changes associated with AMD include micropsia (where objects appear smaller when compared to the unaffected eye) and central scotoma, where peripheral vision is maintained but central vision is lost.

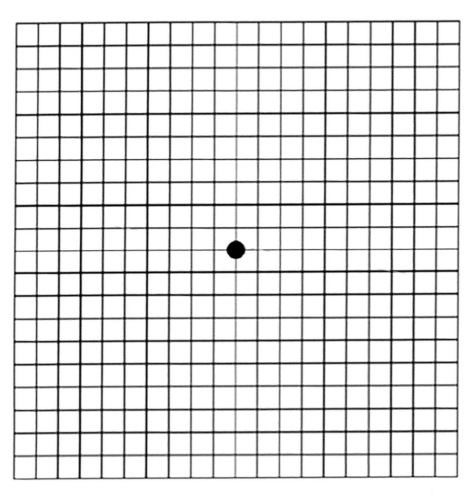

Figure 12.2 An Amsler chart. To use, ask the patient to wear the glasses they use to read and then ask them to cover one eye and look at the central black dot with the uncovered eye. Then ask them to describe any distortion of the lines or dark or blurred areas of the chart. Repeat on the opposite eye.

CLINICAL CONTEXT TIPS

Self-monitoring of dry age-related macular degeneration
Patients diagnosed with dry AMD should be actively encouraged to self-monitor.
The key elements of vision that patients should monitor are:

- Lines that look more wavy than usual
- If there is a central patch of vision missing
- If images look smaller than usual.

For any changes in vision, patients are encouraged to report these changes to their eye care professional and seek advice.

RED FLAG

Patients with wet AMD in their only good eye need urgent management. Discuss the case **same day** with your local eye services to see how soon the patient will be reviewed in the AMD service.

Examination

- Visual acuity
- IOP
- Anterior segment
- Dilated fundus exam.

Investigations

- OCT (see *Chapter 18*)
- FFA (see *Chapter 20*) if available.

Management

Treatment is only currently offered to patients with late AMD (wet active). Disease activity in late AMD (wet active) is determined by:

- A reduction in vision from baseline
- Evidence of active leakage from choroidal neovascularization on OCT or FFA
- Evidence of intraretinal or subretinal haemorrhage.

The current mainstay of treatment is anti-VEGF intravitreal injections, which should be offered within 14 days of referral to the AMD service. Treatment can be monthly or bimonthly depending on the protocol. The agents currently in use in the UK are Eylea (aflibercept), Lucentis (ranibizumab) and Beovu (brolucizumab). Risks associated with anti-VEGF injections include pain, subconjunctival haemorrhage at the site of injection, corneal abrasion, cataract, raised IOP, vitreous floaters, retinal detachment, endophthalmitis (<0.1%) and vision loss.

RED FLAG

A patient presenting with increased pain and redness after an intravitreal injection of anti-VEGF should be assessed **urgently**. These symptoms are most likely due to an iatrogenic corneal abrasion, which usually heals well with topical treatment, but they can also be due to sight-threatening endophthalmitis.

- Assess visual acuity, pupils and intraocular pressure by palpation (instilling a topical ocular anaesthetic may help with this step)
- Anterior segment can be assessed with a pen torch, particularly looking for redness and a hypopyon (see *Figure 10.1*)
- **Immediate referral** to the on-call ophthalmology service.

- Check visual acuity and IOP
- Assess cornea with fluorescein 2% for abrasions or epithelial defects
- Assess anterior chamber for hypopyon or cells
- Perform a dilated fundoscopy to assess the posterior segment
- Confer with local guidelines if endophthalmitis is suspected (increased injection, hypopyon or increased anterior chamber inflammation; see *Section 11.5*).

Both primary and secondary care are instrumental in the education of patients with respect to preventing the progression of their AMD, no matter the grading of disease. Patients should be advised and supported to improve modifiable risk factors such as:
- Smoking – stop
- Body mass index – reduce if appropriate
- Nutrition – ensure diet is rich in leafy green vegetables.

Reaching the ceiling of treatment is a shared decision taken with the patient and their eye care team. Decisions to stop treatment are made when:
- There is no structural improvement (disease activity persists)
- There is no functional improvement (visual acuity continues to decline despite treatment).

Throughout the treatment process, the patient's care team needs to assess the psychosocial impact of the diagnosis of AMD on the patient, and involve support services such as the eye clinic liaison officer (ECLO) and low vision services to help support and advise the patient. Eligibility for certification of visual impairment and DVLA vision standards for driving should also be discussed with the patient (*Figure 12.3*).

Certification of visual impairment criteria

Sight-impaired (partially sighted)

- Group 1: VA between 3/60 and 6/60 Snellen full visual field

- Group 2: VA between 6/60 and 6/24 Snellen with a moderate contraction of visual field

- Group 3: VA between 6/18 Snellen or even better if there is a marked visual field defect, e.g. homonymous hemianopia

Severely sight-impaired

- Group 1: VA of less than 3/60 Snellen (or equivalent)

- Group 2: VA between 3/60 Snellen or better but worse than 6/60 Snellen with constriction of visual field

- Group 3: VA of 6/60 or better with clinically significant contracted field of vision which is functionally impairing the patient, e.g. bitemporal hemianopia

Figure 12.3 Criteria for certification of visual impairment (DOH (2017) Certificate of vision impairment explanatory notes for consultant ophthalmologists and hospital eye clinic staff in England).

CLINICAL CONTEXT TIPS

Charles Bonnet syndrome

Charles Bonnet syndrome arises when patients have visual hallucinations associated with retinal dysfunction and loss of vision, and when there is no other neurological cause for these symptoms. Patients should be asked if they see objects that are not really there, and they should be encouraged to talk about it and given the necessary reassurance and support.

12.3 Retinopathy associated with systemic disease

12.3.1 Diabetic retinopathy

Diabetic retinopathy (DR) causes microvascular changes to the retinal vasculature as a result of the hyperglycaemic state. All patients diagnosed with insulin-dependent or non-insulin-dependent diabetes, and over the age of 12, are invited for community screening for DR once a year (it can be extended to 2 years for low risk patients). Sight-threatening diabetic retinopathy, such as diabetic macular oedema (leaky blood vessels at the macula) or proliferative diabetic retinopathy, should be reviewed in ophthalmology clinic **within 2 weeks if confirmed on diabetic screening**.

History
Ask about:
- Age at diabetes diagnosis

- Diabetic control (ask the patient about their HbA1c)
- History of proteinuria
- Ocular symptoms:
  - reduced vision or loss of vision
  - floaters
  - visual field defect
  - eye pain and redness (*think raised IOP*).

Examination

Assess:

- Visual acuity
- IOP.

Observe for:

- Neovascularization at the iris (perform gonioscopy to look for new blood vessels in the angle)
- Cataract.

Perform dilated fundus exam and observe for:

- Non-proliferative DR:
  - background DR clinical features are:
    - dot and blot haemorrhages (found at the inner nuclear and outer plexiform retinal layers)
    - hard exudates (found in the outer plexiform layer and due to impaired blood–retina barrier)
    - cotton wool spots (caused by ischaemia in the retinal nerve fibre layer)
  - preproliferative DR (*Figure 12.4*) clinical features are:

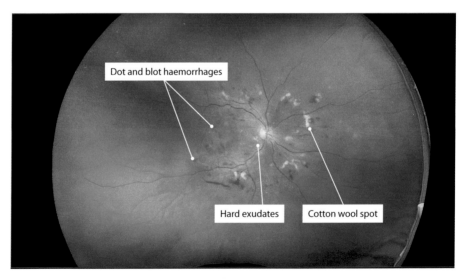

Figure 12.4 Preproliferative diabetic retinopathy.

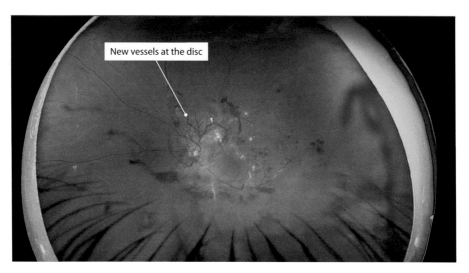

New vessels at the disc

Figure 12.5 Proliferative diabetic retinopathy.

- features of non-proliferative DR, and
- increase in retinal haemorrhages and cotton wool spots
- venous looping and beading
- Proliferative DR:
  - new vessel at the disc (*Figure 12.5*)
  - new vessels elsewhere in the fundus
- Diabetic maculopathy / diabetic macular oedema.

Investigations
- OCT (see *Chapter 18*)
- FFA (see *Chapter 20*) if available.

Management
Diabetic control, as well as control of other cardiovascular risk factors, is important in controlling the ocular sequelae of diabetes. This ischaemic drive caused by diabetes causes the increased secretion of vascular endothelial growth factor (VEGF), which stimulates new vessel growth. The mainstay of treatment of proliferative DR is panretinal photocoagulation (PRP; *Figure 12.6*), which destroys localized areas of retina to reduce the ischaemic drive. For maculopathy, treatment includes laser, intravitreal anti-VEGF and steroid treatments, depending on whether the oedema is fovea-involving and the central retinal thickness on OCT is more than 400 microns (see *Figures 18.3* and *18.4* for OCT appearances of macular oedema).

12.3.2 Hypertensive retinopathy

Hypertensive changes to the retinal vasculature often develop over a period of time, and can occur with chronic hypertension. Patients often do not have any visual symptoms, but findings on dilated fundus examination show early changes including

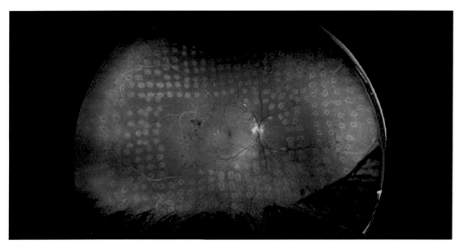

Figure 12.6 Panretinal photocoagulation for proliferative DR.

arteriolar narrowing and silver wiring (sclerotic changes), and with arteriovenous (AV) nipping where the sclerotic arterioles compress the venules where they cross. As it progresses, retinal ischaemia ensues with cotton wool spots and flame haemorrhages at the level of the retinal nerve fibre layer. Retinal vascular occlusion can result from hypertensive retinopathy, which is why blood pressure is one of the modifiable risk factors for retinal vascular occlusion.

Patients with malignant hypertension (blood pressure >200/120mmHg) are more likely to have an accelerated hypertensive retinopathy, with optic disc oedema. These patients are likely to complain of visual disturbances including reduced vision, central scotoma and diplopia if there is microvascular or macrovascular insult to the cranial nerves controlling ocular motility. These patients require **immediate medical referral** for hypertension investigation and control.

12.4 Vascular occlusion

There are four types of vascular occlusion that can occur within the retina:
● Central retinal artery occlusion (CRAO)
● Branch retinal artery occlusion (BRAO)
● Central retinal vein occlusion (CRVO)
● Branch retinal vein occlusion (BRVO).

12.4.1 Retinal artery occlusion

 Patients who present to primary care or A&E with a sudden dramatic reduction in vision should have a **same day referral** to their local emergency eye service.

History
Ask about:
- Age
- Risk factors:
  - diabetes
  - hypertension
  - hyperlipidaemia
  - carotid artery disease
  - cardiac valve disease
  - thrombophilic disorders
  - infection
  - cocaine use (patient <40 years presenting with retinal artery occlusion)
- CRAO:
  - sudden, dramatic drop in vision
  - preceding amaurosis fugax
  - associated pain (*think GCA in those aged over 50*; see *Chapter 14*)
  - associated neurological symptoms:
    - slurred speech
    - limb weakness
    - loss of consciousness
- BRAO:
  - milder loss of vision compared with CRAO
  - no pupillary changes
  - altitudinal visual field defect (*"the top of my vision in my right eye is missing"*).

Examination
Assess:
- Vision
- Colour vision
- IOP
- Pupillary reactions (is there a relative afferent pupillary defect?)
- Temporal tenderness (*think GCA*)
- Dilated fundus exam
  - retinal oedema (pale patches of retina)
  - cherry red spot (*Figure 12.7*)
  - cattle trucking (discontinuity of blood flow in the retinal arteries).

Investigations
- Urgent bloods for CRP and ESR to rule out GCA
- BP and BG.

Management
 Once diagnosis of CRAO has been confirmed on dilated fundus exam (cherry red spot at macula, retinal oedema, arteriolar attenuation; *Figure 12.7*), and no evidence of GCA, a **same day referral** to the local TIA/stroke clinic for further work-up (carotid Doppler, ECG, echocardiogram) is required.

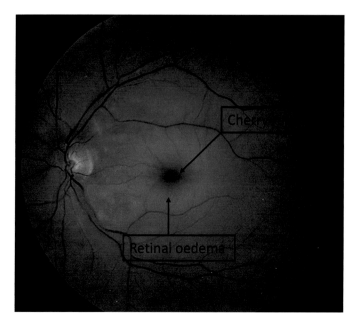

Figure 12.7 Central retinal artery occlusion with cherry red spot over the macula and surrounding retinal oedema.

The main complications of retinal artery occlusion are neovascularization and neovascular glaucoma (although rare compared to this in retinal vein occlusions). Lifestyle modification for atherosclerotic and embolic causes takes a multidisciplinary effort from both the primary care and hospital teams. Patients should be encouraged to control blood pressure, cholesterol and diabetes, and be counselled on smoking cessation where appropriate.

12.4.2 Retinal vein occlusion

 A patient may present to primary care or A&E with an acute change in vision which would warrant a **same day referral** to their local eye service. If the patient has been diagnosed with a retinal vein occlusion (RVO) by their optometrist, same day telephone triage with the local medical retina service is warranted to determine the urgency of review, usually within **2 weeks** (except for patients presenting with features of neovascular glaucoma, who need to be seen same day).

History
Ask about:
- Age
- Pain (should be painless)
- Risk factors:

- o diabetes
- o hypertension
- o hyperlipidaemia
- o carotid artery disease
- o cardiac valve disease
- o blood coagulation disorders (in young patients; either personal or familial)
- o systemic inflammation
- o history of myocardial infarction or stroke
- o use of combined oral contraceptive pill
- o history of sustained, increased intraocular pressure
- CRVO:
  - o sudden, dramatic loss of vision (worse with ischaemic CRVO vs. non-ischaemic CRVO)
- BRVO
  - o milder loss of vision compared with CRVO
  - o altitudinal visual field defect (*"the top of my vision in my right eye is missing"*).

Examination

Assess:
- Vision
- Colour vision
- IOP
- Iris (new vessels at the iris)
- Pupillary reactions (is there a relative afferent pupillary defect?; *think ischaemic RVO*)
- Dilated fundus exam
  - o CRVO: widespread multilaminar retinal haemorrhages (*Figure 12.8*)
  - o BRVO: wedge-shaped retinal haemorrhages
  - o evidence of ischaemia (hard exudates, cotton wool spots)
  - o optic disc oedema
  - o macular oedema.

Investigations

- Blood pressure
- Bloods including FBC, serum glucose and ESR (looking for inflammatory conditions)
- Further blood testing, such as clotting and thrombophilia screen, is dependent on age of the patient and history
- OCT (to assess for macular oedema; see *Chapter 18*)
- FFA (to assess for retinal ischaemia in ischaemic CRVO; see *Chapter 20*).

Management

As with retinal artery occlusions, lifestyle modifications are key to reducing the risk of similar problems in the opposite eye. The main complication of retinal vein occlusions are macular oedema, neovascularization and neovascular glaucoma. Treatment relies on clinical presentation as follows:

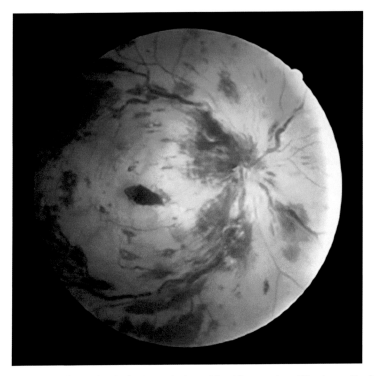

Figure 12.8 Central retinal vein occlusion with widespread multilaminar retinal haemorrhages, optic disc oedema, and retinal vein tortuosity.

- Non-ischaemic CRVO with macular oedema: intravitreal anti-VEGF or steroid should be administered no more than 2–4 weeks from initial presentation.
- Ischaemic CRVO without neovascularization: intravitreal anti-VEGF and steroid can be used for the treatment of macular oedema; however, anti-VEGF should be stopped if there is no response after three injections.
- Ischaemic CRVO with neovascularization: anti-VEGF and PRP dual therapy should be instigated as soon as possible (within 1–2 weeks).
- Neovascular glaucoma: medical and surgical treatment to lower intraocular pressure (see *Section 10.3*), in addition to anti-VEGF and PRP, is necessary to stabilize the disease process. Known as the 90-day glaucoma, it presents with eye pain and raised IOP mainly in patients with ischaemic CRVO.

12.5 Inherited retinal dystrophies

Although rare, some of the more common of the inherited retinal dystrophies seen in an ophthalmology department are described in *Table 12.1*.

Table 12.1 Inherited retinal dystrophies

Disease	Genetics	Pathophysiology	Clinical features	ERG/EOG findings	Further information
Photoreceptor / phototransduction dystrophies					
Retinitis pigmentosa	AD, AR, XL	Photoreceptor dysfunction (rod then cone)	Night blindness Bone spicule retinal pigmentation Arteriolar attenuation Waxy optic disc pallor Posterior subcapsular cataract Myopia Cystoid macular oedema	**ERG:** scotopic responses more affected	25% have syndromic associations
Leber's congenital amaurosis	AR	Dysfunctional phototransduction cascade	Abnormal or absent pupillary responses Hyperopia Initially normal retina Keratoconus Oculodigital syndrome (eye poking) Photophobia Nystagmus Vision 6/400 or less	Extinguished ERG	

Table 12.1 *cont'd*

Disease	Genetics	Pathophysiology	Clinical features	ERG/EOG findings	Further information
Congenital stationary night blindness (CSNB)	AD, AR, XL	**Normal fundus:** AD: dysfunction in rod photo-transduction cascade AR and XL: dysfunction in transmission from photoreceptors to bipolar cells **Abnormal fundus:** Oguchi's disease: dysfunction in the inactivation of rhodopsin in rod phototransduction	Night blindness Nystagmus Myopia Strabismus **Normal fundus:** cCSNB and iCSNB **Abnormal fundus:** Oguchi's disease: golden yellow metallic sheen to fundus, which appears normal after prolonged dark adaptation (Mizuo phenomenon) **Fundus albipunctatus:** discrete uniform white dots/flecks of the retina	**ERG:** AD CSNB: scotopic abnormal AR and XL CSNB: electronegative scotopic ERG with normal a wave and diminished b wave cCSNB: unrecordable scotopic iCSNB: abnormal cone ERGs	
Achromatopsia	AR	Cone dysfunction	Poor vision from birth Poor colour vision from birth Pendular nystagmus Photophobia	**ERG:** Absent cone function; maintained rod function	

Disease	Genetics	Pathophysiology	Clinical features	ERG/EOG findings	Further information
Macular dystrophies					
Stargardt's disease / fundus flavimaculatus	AR: *ABCA4* gene	Accumulation of lipofuscin and A2E throughout the RPE	**Early:** Stargardt's: rapid loss of vision in childhood or adulthood Minimal fundus changes **Late:** Stargardt's: beaten bronze atrophy **Fundus flavimaculatus:** pisciform flecks at the posterior pole; vision preserved	**ERG:** Group 1: macular dysfunction Group 2: macular and generalized cone dysfunction Group 3: macular and generalized cone and rod dysfunction	Dark choroid on FFA
Best's disease	AD: *BEST1* gene	Disruption of ion channels causing RPE dysfunction	**Stage 1:** pre-vitelliform (abnormal EOG only) **Stage 2:** vitelliform ('egg yolk-like lesion') **Stage 3:** pseudohypopyon **Stage 4:** vitelliruptive **Stage 5:** end-stage (atrophy)	**EOG:** reduced Arden ratio (<1.5:1)	
X-linked retinoschisis	XL: *RS1* gene	Disruption of cell-to-cell adhesion	Affected males Onset of symptoms in first decade of life Hyperopia Spoke wheel fovea	**ERG:** reduction in b wave	

Table 12.1 cont'd

Disease	Genetics	Pathophysiology	Clinical features	ERG/EOG findings	Further information
Chorioretinal dystrophies					
Gyrate atrophy	AR: *OAT* gene	Accumulation of ornithine	Myopia Nyctalopia Peripheral vision loss Reduced visual acuity Mid-periphery, patchy RPE and choroidal atrophy	**ERG:** reduced rod responses before cone responses **OCT:** peripheral extensive loss of IS/OS junction Increased plasma ornithine	Highest rate in Finland
Choroideraemia	XL: *CHM* gene Xq21.2	Impairment of transport of proteins from Golgi apparatus to outer segments in photoreceptors	Concentric VF loss Myopia Nyctalopia Reduced visual acuity Mid-periphery, patchy RPE and choroidal atrophy	**ERG:** reduced rod responses before cone responses	
Albinism					
Ocular albinism	XL: *OA1/ GPR143* genes Xp22.3–22.2	Disruption of melanosome transport in pigment cells	Iris transillumination Foveal hypoplasia 'Blond' fundus Nystagmus Refractive error Strabismus	N/A	**OCT:** reduced or absent foveal dip

Disease	Genetics	Pathophysiology	Clinical features	ERG/EOG findings	Further information
Oculocutaneous albinism	AR: chromosomes 9, 11, 15 involved with melanogenesis	Disruption of melanogenesis	Same as above Syndromes: • Hermansky–Pudlak: Puerto Rican ancestry, low platelets • Chediak–Higashi: pyogenic infections	N/A	

AD, autosomal dominant; AR, autosomal recessive; XL, X-linked; cCSNB, complete congenital stationary night blindness; iCSNB, incomplete congenital stationary night blindness.

12.6 Ocular oncology

Uveal melanomas are the most common ocular malignancy, with choroidal melanomas (*Figure 12.9*) accounting for the large majority of these lesions.

History

Patients who present with choroidal melanomas may complain of a variety of visual disturbances including:

- Pain
- Loss of vision
- Visual field defect
- Floaters and flashing lights.

Ask about:

- History of malignancy (breast and lung cancer metastasize to the eye).

Examination

Assess:

- Vision
- IOP
- Anterior segment:
  - sclera (extrascleral extension)
  - iris (new vessels at the iris)
  - lens (for focal cataract due to compression from mass)

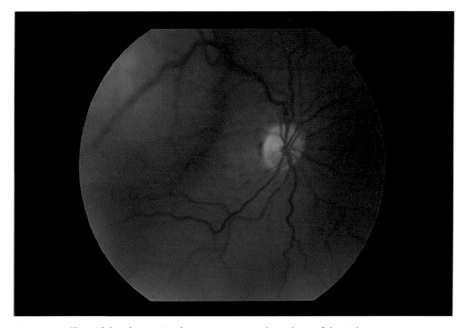

Figure 12.9 Choroidal melanoma in the superotemporal quadrant of the right eye.

- Pupillary reactions
- Dilated fundus exam
  - elevated sub RPE mass which may appear dark brown / black with overlying orange pigment and an associated retinal detachment (compared to a choroidal naevus which is more common, and has a flat, slate-grey appearance with no underlying detachment).

Investigations

Ocular ultrasound will help with the diagnosis, with the features of choroidal melanoma described in *Figure 19.4*.

Suspicion of any uveal tumour warrants referral to one of the Ocular Oncology referral centres in the UK (Glasgow, Liverpool, London and Sheffield). The MOLES (**m**ushroom, **o**range pigment, **l**arge size, **e**nlargement, **s**ubretinal fluid) scoring system will help determine the likelihood of malignancy (see www.rcophth.ac.uk/wp-content/uploads/2021/01/Ocular-Tumour-Refreral-Guidance-August-2022.pdf).

12.7 Investigation of retinal disease: electrodiagnostic testing

The most common and imperative investigation for every medical retina clinic patient is optical coherence tomography (OCT); while fundus fluorescein angiography (FFA) also has a role in assessing retinal ischaemia and neovascularization. *Chapters 18* and *20* discuss the key concepts of OCT and FFA, respectively, and their use in the diagnosis and monitoring of retinal disease. Electrodiagnostic testing such as electroretinogram (ERG) and electrooculogram (EOG) are particularly useful in differentiating between different retinopathies, particularly the inherited retinal diseases.

There are four main components of the full-field ERG (*Figure 12.10*) which illustrates the testing of the rod and cone function separately, as well as in combination. The key features of ERG and EOG and the way they are interpreted are described in *Table 12.2*.

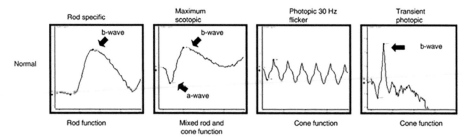

Figure 12.10 Normal full-field ERG tracings showing a and b waves where appropriate. Reproduced from Tsang and Sharma (2018) with permission from Springer-Verlag.

Table 12.2 Features of ERG and EOG testing

Test	Purpose	Interpretation	Examples of disease states where it is abnormal
EOG	RPE and photoreceptor activity	Arden ratio: ● normal >1.80 ● subnormal 1.40–1.80 ● abnormal <1.40	Best's vitelliform macular dystrophy
ERG	Full-field: entire retinal response Pattern ERG: macular function mfERG: summation of electrical potentials from the whole retina with topographical illustration	● a wave: photoreceptors ● b waves: bipolar and Müller cells Scotopic = rods Photopic = cones	Reduced a and b waves ● Rod–cone dystrophy ● Drug toxicity ● Cancer-associated retinopathy ● Ophthalmic artery occlusion Normal a wave, reduced scotopic b wave ● Central retinal vein or artery occlusion ● Congenital stationary night blindness ● Quinine toxicity ● Melanoma-associated retinopathy Abnormal photopic and normal scotopic: ● Cone dystrophy ● Achromatopsia

References and further reading

NICE (2018) NG82: *Age-related Macular Degeneration*.

Royal College of Ophthalmologists (2022) *Referral Pathways for Ocular Tumours*. Available at: www.rcophth.ac.uk/wp-content/uploads/2021/01/Ocular-Tumour-Refreral-Guidance-August-2022.pdf

Royal College of Ophthalmologists (2022) *Retinal Vein Occlusion (RVO)* (Clinical Guidelines). Available at: www.rcophth.ac.uk/wp-content/uploads/2015/07/Retinal-Vein-Occlusion-Guidelines-Executive-Summary-2022.pdf

Tsang, S.H. and Sharma, T. (2018) Electroretinography. In: Tsang, S. and Sharma, T. (eds) *Atlas of Inherited Retinal Diseases*. Advances in Experimental Medicine and Biology, vol 1085, pp. 17–20. Springer. https://doi.org/10.1007/978-3-319-95046-4_5

Chapter 13
Vitreoretinal

13.1 Introduction

Also known as 'surgical retina', vitreoretinal pathology often presents in A&E in the form of 'flashes and floaters'.

In a patient with flashes and floaters, it is important to identify whether the patient simply has:
- Vitreous that's getting older (vitreous syneresis) or a posterior vitreous detachment (PVD: vitreous condensing and pulling away from the retina)
- More emergent pathology: a vitreous haemorrhage (blood in the vitreous), retinal tear (a full-thickness retinal break secondary to the vitreous tugging on the retina) or rhegmatogenous retinal detachment (peeling away of the retina caused by vitreous entering a retinal tear).

Vitreoretinal clinics also treat patients with more chronic conditions such as epiretinal membranes, macular holes and tractional retinal detachments secondary to diabetic retinopathy.

Protocols for treatment differ between vitreoretinal units and so it is crucial to always consult local guidelines.

13.2 Acute presentations

13.2.1 Flashes and floaters

To distinguish between less and more emergent pathology, it is important to understand the process of vitreous degeneration and vitreoretinal traction.

Floaters
The vitreous is the jelly-like substance that fills the posterior segment, in front of the retina (see *Section 2.10* for more detail), which is usually optically clear. As the vitreous ages, it starts to undergo synchysis (liquefaction of the vitreous) and syneresis (breakdown of the collagen arrangement in the vitreous). These processes cause the vitreous gel to degenerate and collagen fibrils clump together, forming the floaters that patients see. These are usually a few semi-translucent floaters but are often described by patients as 'dots', 'webs' or 'worms' in the visual axis that move with the ocular movement. It is important to note that floaters can also be secondary to posterior-segment inflammatory cells in a patient with intermediate or posterior uveitis.

Flashes
Flashes, or photopsia, indicate vitreous tugging or traction on the retina and can be a

symptom of posterior vitreous detachment (which in itself is harmless, but may pave the way for a retinal tear or detachment). Flashes are typically episodes of streaks of light as an arc in the temporal aspect of the vision, often noticed in dim lighting.

Once a retinal tear, vitreous haemorrhage or a rhegmatogenous retinal detachment is excluded (see below), you can reassure your patient that, although annoying, the floaters themselves are harmless. Let the patient know that the floaters represent an ageing process in the gel at the back of the eye and will eventually happen to virtually everyone, and that the floaters will become less apparent over the coming months as the brain neuro-adapts.

RED FLAG

If a patient experiences flashing lights, a sudden increase or shower of floaters, and reduction in vision or curtain-like field defect, an **immediate referral** to local eye services must be done for same day review.

CLINICAL CONTEXT TIPS

What do dark floaters signify?

A sudden onset or shower of dark floaters may indicate a vitreous haemorrhage or retinal tear, both of which should be excluded in any patient presenting with new-onset flashes and floaters.

BOX 13.1: WHO IS A 'HIGH RISK' PATIENT WITH FLASHES AND FLOATERS?

The following patients with flashes and floaters should be referred to an ophthalmologist for further assessment:

- Myope
- Those with a previous history/family history of retinal tear or retinal detachment (i.e. something that's needed retinal laser or intraocular vitreoretinal surgery)
- Those following trauma or intraocular surgery
- Any with connective tissue disorders (Marfan or Ehlers–Danlos syndromes)
- Those with a sudden worsening of symptoms – sudden shower/explosion of floaters, increase in photopsia, dark curtain progressing across field.

Posterior vitreous detachment

PVD is the physiological, age-related process of the vitreous jelly separating from the retina. Although the majority of the time it does not cause any adverse pathology, it can cause a retinal tear and lead to a retinal detachment.

Once a retinal tear, vitreous haemorrhage or a rhegmatogenous retinal detachment is excluded on dilated fundus exam you can reassure your patient that, although annoying, the floaters themselves are harmless. Let the patient know that the floaters represent an ageing process in the gel at the back of the eye and will eventually happen to virtually everyone, and that the floaters will become less apparent over the coming months as the brain neuro-adapts.

Patients with flashing lights and floaters must be reviewed within 24 hours (they can see their optometrist). High risk patients (see *Box 13.1*) need referral to ophthalmology department **within 24 hours**. Patients with a visual field defect need **same day** ophthalmology review.

All patients require a dilated fundus exam to exclude vitreous haemorrhage, retinal tear and retinal detachment. Once excluded, the patient is reassured and discharged, with the safety net to seek urgent medical attention if there are any red flag symptoms. High risk patients who are symptomatic (but with no vitreous pigment / haemorrhage, retinal tear or break seen) should undergo a repeated dilated fundal exam in 4 weeks, with verbal and written advice to return earlier should they have any worsening of their symptoms in the meanwhile.

CLINICAL CONTEXT TIP

What does flashing lights in both eyes signify?
Simultaneous bilateral flashing phenomenon is unlikely to represent ophthalmic pathology. It can represent migraine with aura (especially if associated with patterns) or cerebral vascular issues such as vertebrobasilar insufficiency.

Retinal tear

Although most patients have an uncomplicated PVD, in a minority of patients the PVD will cause a full-thickness retinal tear. This usually occurs in the early stages because once the vitreous is more fully detached from the retina, the major 'traction' effect on the retina is released. Symptoms may include a sudden increase in flashes or floaters or a change in their morphology: countless dark dots rather than the odd large floater. Tears usually start as a 'horseshoe tear' (*Figure 13.1*), but if the entire 'plug' of retinal tissue comes away and is avulsed in the vitreous, this is known as an 'operculated' tear.

Urgently refer patients to ophthalmology (same day or, if presenting overnight, first thing the following morning).

Exclude retinal detachment subsequent to tear. Management options include laser retinopexy (*Figures 13.2* and *13.3*) or cryoretinopexy for horseshoe tears. In some units treatment is also given for operculated tears, especially if symptomatic or history of retinal detachment in fellow eye.

CLINICAL CONTEXT TIPS

When is cryoretinopexy used?

Cryoretinopexy can be advantageous in certain cases, e.g. if the tear is too anterior for laser retinopexy, but carries a higher risk of epiretinal membrane formation, proliferative vitreoretinopathy and choroidal detachment.

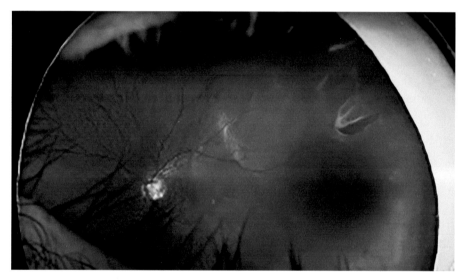

Figure 13.1 Wide-field colour fundus photograph of the left eye, showing a superotemporal horseshoe tear (U-tear); fluid has started to collect under the tear progressing to a retinal detachment.

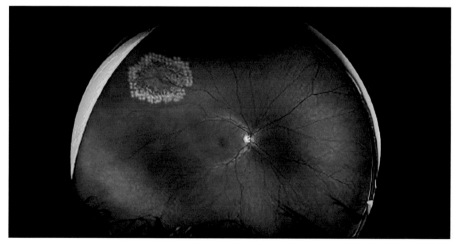

Figure 13.2 Wide-field colour fundus photo of right eye, depicting a superotemporal retinal horseshoe tear, treated with rows of laser barrage (white scars).

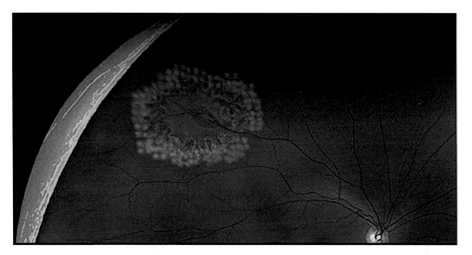

Figure 13.3 Higher magnification view of treated retinal tear (laser retinopexy).

BOX 13.2: CONSENTING FOR RETINOPEXY

Benefits: prevents vision loss from retinal detachment
Risks:
- Sight-threatening from: failure (retinal detachment) or macular burns
- Worse vision from: epiretinal membrane, cystoid macular oedema, inflammation, raised intraocular pressure, vitreous haemorrhage.

Retinal detachment

If fluid escapes through the retinal tear and causes the retina to peel off (like wallpaper peeling off a wall), this is a rhegmatogenous retinal detachment (*Figure 13.4*).

The patient will notice a shadow or curtain-like field defect progressing over their vision (in the opposite area to where the detachment is, i.e. superior field defects indicate inferior detachments). Central visual field being affected indicates that the macula is involved. Due to the effect of gravity when upright, superior detachments are more imminently sight-threatening because they can progress downward to affect the macula more quickly.

 If a retinal detachment is diagnosed by an optometrist, refer patients **same day** to ophthalmology (if presenting overnight, first thing the following morning).

 Locate the tear(s) and refer to local vitreoretinal team for surgical repair.

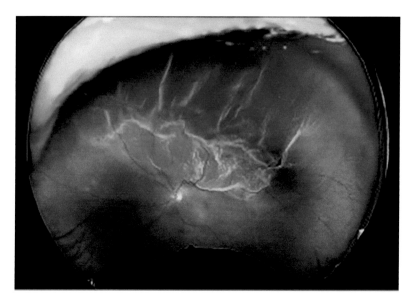

Figure 13.4 Wide-field colour fundus photo of left eye. A superotemporal retinal tear has led to a superior retinal detachment, affecting the superior macula.

Management

The principle for retinal detachment repair is to find the retinal tear(s), seal them (with chorioretinal scarring using laser or cryotherapy) and then plug them (eliminate the traction using tamponades or explants).

Repair options include vitrectomy with intraocular gas (where the patient postures to ensure the bubble is moved towards the area of the break; gas eventually dissolves) or oil (which needs to be removed) as an internal tamponade, or scleral buckling as an external explant (especially in patients without PVD, shallow inferior detachments and young phakic patients).

Vitreoretinal surgery risks include loss of vision or worse vision from bleeding, infection, raised IOP, inflammation, recurrent retinal detachments or tears, and eventual cataract.

Post-operative follow-up care for these patients includes counselling, IOP and inflammation control, ensuring the retina remains attached, and monitoring for cataract in patients who have had a vitrectomy. Patients should be counselled to always monitor both eyes for red flag symptoms such as:

- Persistent flashing lights
- Sudden increase or shower of floaters
- Reduction in vision or curtain-like field defect.

Vitreous haemorrhage

Blood in the vitreous jelly can cause a sudden shower of dark floaters or profound, acute, painless vision loss if the bleed is dense. This is usually a bleed from a retinal blood vessel, either:

- A native vessel during a PVD, retinal tear or detachment
- A new abnormal blood vessel in conditions such as diabetic retinopathy or retinal vein occlusion where retinal ischaemia stimulates abnormal, fragile neovascularization.

Your main job is to identify the cause of vitreous haemorrhage and exclude retinal tear and detachment as emergent causes.

 In a patient presenting with new onset dark floaters, refer patients **same day** to ophthalmology (if presenting overnight, first thing the following morning).

 Exclude retinal tear and retinal detachment as emergent causes – this may require B-scanning if poor fundal view.

The causes of vitreous haemorrhage are listed in *Box 13.3*.

In patients with no obvious cause, a dense fundus-obscuring vitreous haemorrhage is considered secondary to a hidden retinal tear (or detachment). Patients require urgent vitreoretinal surgery to clear the blood and treat any retinal tear/detachment. Rapid self-resolution is rare, and delaying surgery can worsen outcomes.

Diabetic patients with no previous history of diabetic retinopathy should be discussed with the vitreoretinal team to plan management (examination of the fellow eye can give clues). A patient with known proliferative diabetic retinopathy must also be discussed with the vitreoretinal team, who may watchfully wait for the haemorrhage to clear, or plan for early vitrectomy plus panretinal photocoagulation.

> ### BOX 13.3: CAUSES OF VITREOUS HAEMORRHAGE
>
> Proliferative diabetic retinopathy (most common), retinal tear, haemorrhagic PVD, retinal detachment, retinal vein occlusion, age-related macular degeneration, retinal macro-aneurysm, sickle cell retinopathy, trauma, tumour.

History

The aim of history-taking in a patient with flashing lights or floaters is to try to differentiate between low risk pathology (vitreous syneresis/PVD) and high risk pathology (vitreous haemorrhage, retinal tear or detachment). In a non-ophthalmic clinical setting, it will provide information to make an appropriate referral.

Ask about:
- Onset of symptoms
- Type of floaters: number, character (a few semi-translucent floaters indicate vitreous syneresis or PVD, whereas too many to count or a dark shower indicates a vitreous haemorrhage or retinal tear), and whether they move with ocular movement
- Area of photopsia: typically a temporal arc noticed in dim light
- Any 'shadow' or 'curtain'-like field defect (*think retinal detachment*; if progressed to the centre of the vision this indicates macular involvement)
- Any reduction in visual acuity

- Exclude migraine symptoms (e.g. bilateral patterns of colours, heatlines, headache history)
- Exclude loss of vision from other causes:
  - a main complaint of **profound acute** *vision loss* (either total or part of field, as opposed to a **progressive shadow** / *dark curtain*) is unlikely to be related to vitreoretinal traction; consider retinal vascular occlusion, optic neuropathy and always rule out GCA symptoms
- Past ocular history, particularly retinal conditions (e.g. diabetic retinopathy, RVO, any condition where retinal/choroidal neovascularization can develop)
- Past medical history (i.e. anaesthetic considerations, if applicable, for potential surgery)
- Risk factors for vitreoretinal pathology in past medical history, past ocular history and family history:
  - refractive status: higher risk if myopic
  - personal/family history of connective tissue disorders (e.g. Marfan's) or syndromes (e.g. Stickler's)
  - previous history/family history of retinal tear or retinal detachment (i.e. something that's required retinal laser, cryotherapy or intraocular vitreoretinal surgery)
  - preceding ocular trauma or surgery.

CLINICAL CONTEXT TIPS

How to refer high risk patients with flashing lights and floaters
A patient with new floaters/flashes with any risk factors would be classified as 'high risk' and should be examined, **preferably same day**, by an ophthalmic clinician. Some areas have urgent-care optometrists who are qualified to examine the peripheral retina and can refer on to the ophthalmology department if there is any concern, whereas in other areas this assessment would have to be undertaken in the ophthalmology department.

This history can all be undertaken in primary care or A&E and will provide enough information to manage the patient prior to ophthalmology referral. In the ophthalmology clinic, this history will help determine if this is likely to be syneresis/PVD or something more emergent.

Examination

Assess:
- Visual acuity
- Pupil examination.

- IOP
- History of cataract surgery
- Dilated fundus exam:
  - separation of the posterior hyaloid membrane from the retina – you may see the vitreous just posterior to the lens with its posterior

membrane visible, then a dark 'empty' black space just posterior to that. You may also notice a Weiss ring: the attachment of the vitreous to the disc (this is a strong area of vitreous attachment to the fundus and seeing the Weiss ring indicates an essentially 'complete' PVD)

o   pigment (tobacco dust / Shafer's sign) or red blood cells in the vitreous: indicates that there has been a tear in the retina. Not seeing pigment is reassuring, but not necessarily indicative that there is no tear!

o   a full peripheral fundal examination using wide-field lenses, 3-mirror lenses and indirect ophthalmoscopy with indentation to visualize breaks / tears (most commonly superior–temporal) or retinal detachment; in 50% of cases where a break is visualized, there are more elsewhere

o   check for predisposing lesions such as peripheral vitreoretinal degenerations (lattice, round holes)

o   if a detachment is seen, assess for signs of chronicity: demarcation line, cysts, proliferative vitreoretinopathy

o   if vitreous haemorrhage is seen, check for underlying conditions: retinal haemorrhages with neovascularization.

Investigations

Ancillary testing is only needed if it is a difficult examination or if there is doubt of the diagnosis. Optical coherence tomography (OCT) of the posterior hyaloid membrane can be helpful in diagnosing PVD (though this can be confused for the premacular bursa). Ocular ultrasound can be used if there is a poor view of the fundus (due to cataract or vitreous haemorrhage). If in doubt ask the vitreoretinal team for help.

CLINICAL CONTEXT TIPS

● Floaters (± flashes) are common and usually represent vitreous syneresis ± posterior vitreous detachment; these conditions are usually harmless

● High risk patients or those with symptoms suggestive of retinal tear, vitreous haemorrhage or retinal detachment must be seen urgently (same day or if presenting overnight, first thing next morning).

13.3 Chronic presentations

13.3.1 Epiretinal membranes

An epiretinal membrane is a thickened, semi-translucent membrane overlying the macula and can be associated with retinal vascular tortuosity. This is usually idiopathic and related to PVD (a proliferation of retinal glial cells from the posterior hyaloid membrane population or those that have migrated through defects in the internal limiting membrane). It can also be secondary to retinal surgery or retinopexy, trauma, previous retinal tear, retinal vascular occlusions or chronic inflammation. Typical patients are female, in their 50s, with symptoms of metamorphopsia or scotoma, reduced visual acuity and monocular diplopia; although patients can be surprisingly asymptomatic.

Routine referral to ophthalmology is indicated for symptomatic patients, where secondary causes should be ruled out and a macular OCT scan to highlight the epiretinal membrane should be performed. Most cases remain stable from the time of presentation, so asymptomatic cases can be reassured. If symptomatic (visual acuity <6/12 and distortion), **refer routinely** to the vitreoretinal service to consider surgery (vitrectomy + membrane peel ± internal limiting membrane peel ± intraocular gas). Patients should understand that improvement may be slow and not full, especially if there is concurrent macular pathology, lower pre-operative visual acuity and long duration of symptoms.

13.3.2 Macular holes

A macular hole is a small gap opening up at the fovea, usually secondary to traction from the vitreous during the process of a PVD. As the vitreous is attached more firmly to the macula, it can be pulled and stretched as the jelly detaches (traction), and in combination with tangential traction from retinal pigment epithelial / glial cells can lead to a macular hole. Secondary causes can be trauma, previous laser, retinal detachment or cystoid macular oedema. Typical patients are female, over 50 with unilateral (or, in around one-third of cases, bilateral) impaired central vision, scotoma or metamorphopsia. They can be asymptomatic if it is affecting the non-dominant eye.

For symptomatic patients **routine or fast-track referral** to the vitreoretinal clinic is indicated (same day urgent review is not warranted). Clinical examination includes ruling out secondary causes and performing macular OCT to help stage the hole. Vitreomacular adhesion (perifoveal vitreous detachment, with attached vitreous at the macula) and traction (PVD with anatomical distortion of the fovea) can be observed because these usually spontaneously resolve with a full PVD over time. Full-thickness macular hole patients can be treated with surgery (vitrectomy + internal limiting membrane peel + intraocular gas ± patient posturing).

References and further reading

Knott, L. (2021) *Retinal Detachment: causes, signs and treatment*. Available at: https://patient.info/eye-care/visual-problems/retinal-detachment

Royal College of Ophthalmologists (2022) Patient information booklets. Available at: www.rcophth.ac.uk/patients/patient-information-booklets

Chapter 14
Neuro-ophthalmology

14.1 Introduction

Neuro-ophthalmology describes the connection between the eyes and the brain. Neuro-ophthalmologists are sub-specialists involved in the diagnosis and management of patients with a subset of signs and symptoms attributed to any condition that affects the visual pathway; this includes the optic nerves, optic tract, chiasm, post chiasm structures, as well as the extraocular muscles and the cranial nerves.

In primary care and A&E, patients with conditions affecting the visual pathway typically present with associated neurological signs and symptoms, as well as:
- Headache
- Blurred vision or loss of vision
- Double vision (diplopia).

The aim here is to obtain a thorough history and perform an examination, including of the neurological system, to ascertain where is most appropriate to refer the patient, and how quickly. Assessment of visual symptoms can provide key diagnostic clues, but it is important to appreciate that **not all patients with visual symptoms require referral to ophthalmology**; they could have a neurological condition (e.g. stroke, myasthenia gravis crisis, pituitary apoplexy) that requires **immediate neuroimaging and referral to the neurological team**.

Patients with neuro-ophthalmology complaints that present to ophthalmology require a complete ophthalmology assessment, with dilated fundoscopy and ancillary testing such as perimetry for visual field assessment (see *Chapter 17*), and the use of optical coherence tomography (see *Chapter 18*) imaging to aid in diagnosis and for documentation.

14.2 Basic visual pathway anatomy

The visual pathway incorporates the retina, optic nerve, optic chiasm, optic tract, lateral geniculate bodies, optic radiations and visual cortex (*Figure 14.1*).

The retina gathers information that is processed by the brain as an image. It is roughly divided into temporal and nasal retina, with the temporal retina viewing the nasal visual field and the nasal retina viewing the temporal retinal field. The fibres from the retina coalesce to form the optic nerve which exits the posterior eye and enters the optic foramen and the optic canal, situated in the sphenoid bone. The optic nerve has four parts: the intraocular, intraorbital, intracanalicular and intracranial.

The two optic nerves combine posterior and superior to the pituitary gland to form the optic chiasm. It is at this point that half of the fibres from the nasal retina of each eye cross to join the temporal fibres from the contralateral eye to form the optic tract (e.g. the left nasal fibres join the right temporal fibres to form the right optic tract).

The optic tracts course posteriorly, and the majority of the fibres synapse in the lateral geniculate bodies (located in the thalamus and serving as the major relay centre for the visual pathway). The rest of the fibres go on to other nuclei to form the parasympathetic innervation pathway of the pupil.

From the lateral geniculate bodies, the optic tracts become the optic radiations, which course posteriorly to terminate in the primary visual cortex, situated in the occipital lobe.

Knowledge of the visual pathway is key to understanding the visual field defects (VFDs) patients can present with, and so will guide referral and neuroimaging required.

14.3 Neuro-ophthalmology examination

Aside from a thorough history, any patient presenting with visual disturbances, with or without other neurological features, requires a thorough examination (including a neurological examination; see *Table 14.1*). The key features of the neuro-ophthalmology examination include visual acuity (best corrected with any glasses or contact lens the patient may wear), colour vision (looking for red desaturation), the swing torch test to assess for relative afferent pupillary defect (RAPD), confrontation field testing to determine any peripheral or central visual field defects, and assessment of eye movements. Each element of these examinations can be performed in primary care, A&E, and in the ophthalmology department.

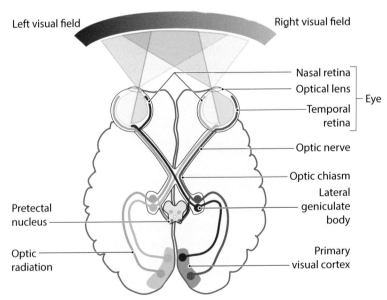

Figure 14.1 Visual pathway. Reproduced under a CC BY-SA 4.0 licence from https://en.wikipedia. org/wiki/Visual_system#/media/File:Human_visual_pathway.svg. Author: Miquel Perello Nieto.

Vision (see *Section 2.2*)

- If a Snellen chart (see *Appendix 1*) is not available to formally test visual acuity, then simply standing in front of the patient (6 metres away from them) and asking them how many fingers you are holding up, is a quick and efficient way to crudely assess if the vision is equal in both eyes – or a mobile phone app can be used.
- Do not forget to ask the patient if they wear glasses or contact lenses.
- In the ophthalmology department, a formal visual acuity test should be performed with an age-appropriate chart (e.g. Snellen, HOTV or Cardiff cards).

Colour vision (see *Section 2.2*)

- Colour vision is formally assessed using Ishihara plates, but if these aren't available in a primary care or A&E setting, then showing the patient a red object monocularly (e.g. the cover of a bottle of eye drops or a red pen) can help determine if there is a difference in colour saturation between the two eyes (*think optic neuropathy*).

Pupils (see *Section 2.8*)

- Observe the size of pupils in both bright and dim light – is there any difference?
- Use a ruler to document the size in millimetres, in both bright and dim light
- Is there any difference in colour of the iris (i.e. heterochromia)?

Swing torch test (see *Figure 2.20*)

- The technique for this is as follows:
  - room light should be dim
  - provide a distant target for the patient to look at
  - swing the torch between each eye, resting for 2–3 seconds on each eye; a normal response is constriction each time the light is shone on either eye
  - if there were a **left** RAPD:
    - illuminate the right pupil (for 3 seconds) – both pupils should constrict
    - quickly illuminate the left pupil (for 3 seconds) – both pupils would dilate
    - swing back to illuminate the right pupil – both pupils should constrict
    - swing back to illuminate the left pupil – both pupils would dilate.

Confrontation field testing

- This test is very useful to determine gross visual field defects
- Start by asking the patient *"is there any part of your field of view missing?"*
- The test can be performed in two parts:
  - Part 1
    - ask the patient to keep focused on your nose, then ask them to cover one of their eyes
    - ask them *"does any part of my face appear missing or blurred?"*
    - repeat for the opposite eye
  - Part 2
    - sit 1 metre away from the patient
    - ask the patient to cover one eye, and you cover the opposite eye (if they cover their right, you cover your left)
    - ask the patient to focus on your uncovered eye

- hold your arms out midway between you and the patient and in the mid-periphery of your field of view
- ask the patient to count how many fingers you are holding up
- repeat this for all four quadrants of the field of view (superotemporal, superonasal, inferotemporal, inferonasal).

Ocular alignment and movements

- Ocular misalignment (strabismus or squint) can readily be assessed using observation, the pen torch and corneal reflex (see *Figure 15.4*)
- The cardinal eye movements were described in *Figure 2.8*, and can be assessed by asking the patient to look in these positions of gaze, with any limitations in movement observed in ductions (monocular eye movements) and versions (binocular eye movements)

- Two elements of eye movements can be assessed and give clues to pathology: **saccades** (fast eye movement to fixate an object onto the fovea) and **pursuit** (slow eye movement to maintain a fixed object on the fovea) are useful in assessing for brainstem or cerebellar pathology:
  - **saccades**
    - tested by observing how quickly a patient can fixate onto a target
    - hold up two fixation targets (fist on one side and index finger on the other side)
    - ask the patient to *"look at my fist"*, pause for 2 seconds, then ask them to *"look at my finger"*
    - this can repeated in the horizontal and vertical planes
  - **pursuit**
    - ask the patient to *"follow my finger without moving your head"*.

Further examination in primary care can be continued by using a pen torch to assess the anterior segment of the eye and a direct ophthalmoscope to determine if there is any optic disc or macular pathology.

Further neurological assessment of the limbs and cranial nerves can also be performed, whether it is in primary care, A&E or the ophthalmology department, to further delineate any additional neurological concerns of the patient's presentation (see *Table 14.1*).

CLINICAL CONTEXT TIPS

How to perform direct ophthalmoscopy

This is a skill that requires practice, including trying to find a direct ophthalmoscope in a busy A&E! In order to visualize the optic disc, as well as the macula, use the following steps:

1. Switch on the ophthalmoscope to check that it is working.
2. Use the aperture dial to set the medium aperture – this is used to view the fundus through a non-dilated pupil in a dark room.
3. Position the patient and ask them to look at a distant target.

4. Dim the room lights.
5. For the **right** eye of the patient, use your **right** hand to hold the direct ophthalmoscope and use your **right** eye to look through the viewing window of the instrument.
6. Find the red reflex.
7. Move closer to the patient, keeping the red reflex in view.
8. Warn the patient (if conscious), that you will be getting quite close to them.
9. Keep viewing through the nasal aspect of the pupil, and use the dioptre dial to bring the fundus into view (if the patient is myopic, turn the dial to the 'red' numbers, and if the patient is hyperopic, turn the dial to the 'green' numbers).
10. Assess the disc for 'cup, colour and contour' to determine any swelling. Also remember to look for any haemorrhages.
11. Also look more temporally to view the macula / fovea.

A dilated fundus exam is an important part of any neuro-ophthalmology examination, and this is normally performed once the patient is reviewed in the ophthalmology department. Fundus examination for neuro-ophthalmology complaints is useful for identifying optic disc oedema / swelling (*Figure 14.2*) or pallor, as well as evidence of central retinal artery occlusion (see *Figure 12.7*).

CLINICAL CONTEXT TIPS

Papilloedema vs. optic disc oedema
The term 'papilloedema' is defined as optic disc swelling caused by increased intracranial pressure. If there is swelling of the optic disc due to other causes, it is described as optic disc oedema.

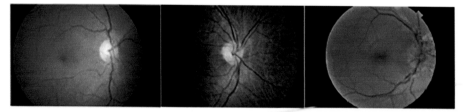

Figure 14.2 Optic disc (left to right: normal; optic disc with mild oedema and with slight blunting of the temporal border of the disc, and obscuration of the small disc vessels; gross optic disc oedema with blunting of the optic disc margin, obliteration of the optic cup, and haemorrhages.

Table 14.1 Brief neurological examination

Upper and lower limb	Cranial nerve	Cerebellar
Assess gait (*"Walk in a straight line". Is the patient waddling or falling over?*) Assess tone (*passively flex and extend at the elbow and knee; is it stiff?*) Assess power (*"Stop me from pushing your shoulders down, stop me from pulling your knees straight"*) Assess sensation (*"Is any part of your face or body numb?"*) Assess reflexes (*knee and elbow*)	CN I (olfactory) • Any changes to smell CN II (optic nerve) • Any changes to vision • Colour vision • Pupils CN III (oculomotor nerve) • Assess eye position and eye movements CN IV (trochlear nerve) • Assess eye position and eye movements CN V (trigeminal) • Check corneal sensation • Check facial sensation • *Pretend to chew* CN VI (abducens) • Assess eye position and eye movements CN VII (facial) • *"Smile"* • *"Show me your teeth"* CN VIII (vestibulocochlear) • Any changes to hearing CN IX (glossopharyngeal) • *"Say Ahh"* • Look for uvula elevation • *"Swallow"* CN X (vagus) • *"Swallow"* CN XI (spinal accessory) • *"Shrug your shoulders"* CN XII (hypoglossal) • *"Stick your tongue out"*	Assess ataxia Assess speech (*"Say 'baby hippopotamus'"*) Check for nystagmus (rapid eye movements) Check for coordination (*"Touch your nose, now touch my finger as fast as you can"*)

14.4 Headache

Patients with headache form a large proportion of primary care and A&E presentations. Headache in the context of ophthalmology may occur in acute angle closure (*Section 10.3*), and in the context of neuro-ophthalmology: papilloedema, third nerve palsy due to a ruptured aneurysm or giant cell arteritis.

Headache may be associated with visual disturbances such as blurred vision, loss of vision or diplopia. All the structures in the head can cause a headache, so it is important to identify the location of headache (*"show me where your head hurts"*); the following other aspects should also be established when looking into the patient's history to determine the cause of the headache:

- Age
- Site (is it frontal or occipital, or is it coming from the eye or paranasal sinuses?)
- Onset (was it sudden (e.g. in a ruptured aneurysm) or insidious?)
- What kind of pain is it (sharp, dull)?
- Does the pain stay in one place?
- Any associated symptoms indicating a neurological rather than ophthalmic cause?
  - any loss of consciousness or seizure? (if so, was it witnessed?)
  - systemic stroke symptoms:
    - any limb weakness or loss of sensation?
    - any facial droop?
    - any slurred speech?
- Any visual disturbance?
  - blurred vision
  - loss of vision (*think GCA*)
  - diplopia (*think nerve palsy or papilloedema*)
  - transient visual obscurations (*think raised intracranial pressure and papilloedema*)
  - was there bilateral visual disturbance – especially colours, patterns or heatwaves – preceding the headache? (*think migraine*)
- Does anything help or make the pain worse?
- Is it giant cell arteritis (GCA)? (consider this in patients aged over 50 with new onset headache)
  - jaw claudication (*"have you been having pain whilst chewing?"*)
  - temporal tenderness (*"have you found your head tender when combing your hair or lying on a pillow at night?"*)
  - weight loss (*"have you found yourself not being able to eat as much or have you lost weight?; are your clothes more loose than before?"*)
  - girdle pain (*"have you had new pain in your hips or shoulders?"*)
  - history of rheumatoid arthritis / polymyalgia rheumatica
  - visual changes (*"do you have blurred vision or loss of vision?; are you seeing two of anything?"*)
- Is it raised intracranial pressure (especially in a young female patient with a high body mass index)?
  - *"is your headache worse in the morning?"*
  - *"is your headache worse when you bend down or strain?"*
  - tinnitus (*"do you have any ringing or buzzing in your ears?"*)
  - transient visual obscurations (*"have you had any episodes where your vision goes black for a few seconds and then returns?"*)
  - any central loss of vision or enlarged blind spot?
- Past medical history
  - diabetes
  - hypertension
  - previous stroke or heart attack

- cancer diagnosis (*think intracranial metastasis*)
    - pro-thrombotic state (previous DVT)
    - pregnancy (remember pre-eclampsia can present as a headache)
- Medications
- Social history
    - smoking
    - alcohol
    - illicit drugs
    - coffee intake (did they recently give up coffee after drinking more than five cups a day for many years?).

14.5 Blurred vision

Blurred vision can present with disease of the eye, the optic nerve, the optic chiasm and the retrochiasmal pathway, as well as arising from non-organic causes (a diagnosis of exclusion following thorough ophthalmic assessment).

The following are key aspects of the history for a patient presenting with blurred vision that can be used in both primary care / A&E and ophthalmology settings (note the overlap between this and the history for headache presentation; see *Section 14.4*):

- Age
- One eye or both eyes? (both more likely to be a neurological cause)
- Onset (fast or gradual? Gradual reduction in vision can be due to cataracts, dry age-related macular degeneration or glaucoma, but in a neuro-ophthalmic context is likely to be due to a slowly progressing visual field defect)
- Which part of the vision is blurred? (total vision, part, central)
- Is it better, worse or the same over time; does it fluctuate?
- Associated symptoms:
    - any headache
    - any loss of consciousness
    - any limb weakness or loss of sensation
    - any facial droop
    - any slurred speech
    - any ocular or orbital pain
    - any diplopia
- Is it typical acute optic neuritis?
    - age under 45, typically Caucasian female patient
    - rapid unilateral drop in vision, worsening over days, and reduced colour vision
    - visual field defect (central scotoma; see *Section 14.8*)
    - pain on eye movement but eye not red
    - symptoms worse in heat / on exercise (Uhthoff's phenomenon)
    - history of multiple sclerosis.

CLINICAL CONTEXT TIPS

What is optic neuropathy?
Optic nerve pathology can be referred to as 'optic neuropathy'. This can broadly be due either to reduced blood supply (ischaemic optic neuropathy, described below) or inflammation (optic neuritis – which in turn can be demyelinating, inflammatory, infective (when acute), or compressive / infiltrative (when gradual)).

CLINICAL CONTEXT TIPS

Typical or atypical optic neuritis?
'Typical' refers to inflammation due to demyelination and is associated with multiple sclerosis, with the above symptoms but generally no optic disc swelling on examination. These should be referred urgently to ophthalmology for confirmation of the diagnosis, where a neurology referral and MRI brain and orbits with contrast can then be requested to assess for demyelination and help prognosticate for multiple sclerosis. The natural history of the condition means visual acuity usually recovers after around 3–5 weeks.

'Atypical' optic neuritis is due to rarer syndromes (MOG-antibody demyelination and neuromyelitis optica) and can have a more profound, bilateral visual loss, less pain and will have disc swelling on examination. These patients, on referral to ophthalmology, would be worked up with blood tests (inflammatory and infective screen, MOG and aquaporin 4 antibodies), neurology input and need to receive urgent high dose intravenous steroids.

- Is it acute anterior ischaemic optic neuropathy (AION – an interruption of the blood supply to the optic nerve)? (see *Red flag* box below)
  - arteritic (caused by inflammation of arteries):
    - GCA symptoms, especially if over 50 years (see above)
    - transient loss of vision episodes preceding acute loss of vision
    - bilateral (starts in one eye and goes to the other eye)
  - non-arteritic (caused by atherosclerosis of arteries):
    - age over 55 years
    - vasculopath (diabetes, hypertension, high cholesterol, smoker)
    - unilateral
    - visual field defect (altitudinal, see *Section 14.8*)
- Is it amaurosis fugax? (see *Red flag* box below)
  - any age
  - monocular transient loss of vision
  - recovery within seconds to minutes
  - *"like a curtain coming down over my vision"*
  - vasculopath suggesting carotid stenosis

- o cocaine use
- o must rule out any GCA symptoms
- Past medical history
  - o diabetes
  - o hypertension
  - o previous stroke or heart attack
  - o cancer diagnosis (think intracranial metastasis)
  - o pro-thrombotic state (previous DVT)
  - o pregnancy (remember pre-eclampsia can present as a headache)
- Medications
- Social history
  - o smoking
  - o alcohol
  - o illicit drugs
  - o coffee intake (did they recently give up coffee after drinking more than five cups a day for many years?)

In primary care or A&E, it is often difficult to decipher any ocular disease of the posterior segment. Therefore any patient presenting with acute blurred vision and any

RED FLAG

Arteritic (GCA) vs. non-arteritic AION

GCA is a life-threatening vasculitic disease that can rapidly lead to permanent vision loss and other morbidity (stroke, aortic aneurysm). Any patient with a suspicion of GCA must be commenced on high dose systemic steroids, and urgent platelets, ESR and CRP should be taken. As well as examining as described in *Section 14.3*, check for temporal artery tenderness and pulsatility. The optic disc in arteritic ischaemic optic neuropathy is swollen with chalky pallor and can have haemorrhages. If vision is already compromised, the patient will likely need admitting for IV methylprednisolone (along with gastric and bone protection). The diagnosis is confirmed with ultrasound or urgent temporal artery biopsy (although treatment should be started empirically, prior to acquiring these).

Each local hospital will have different guidelines for the referral of suspected GCA patients (e.g. rheumatology would be the first referral point if there are no ocular signs, whilst ophthalmology / neuro-ophthalmology would be the first referral point if there are ocular signs). Become familiar with your local guidelines for GCA, as these patients require same day referral to prevent blindness or systemic morbidity from the disease.

NAION patients should have blood pressure, lipid levels (and vasculitis screen if under the age of 50) checked as well as ESR/CRP to rule out GCA. Management is conservative – once confirmed that this is definitely non-arteritic, the patient should be counselled to improve their cardiovascular risk factors.

symptoms mentioned above should have a **same day referral** to an ophthalmology service for a complete work-up, unless there are other neurological symptoms that point to a referral to neurology or neurosurgery in the first instance. Of course, first discussing any visual complaints with your local ophthalmology department can help formulate a solid referral plan.

RED FLAG

Amaurosis fugax

Transient monocular vision loss should be treated as a transient ischaemic attack (TIA) of the eye until proven otherwise. In these cases, the patient should have a same day referral to the TIA/stroke clinic because patients experiencing amaurosis fugax are at high risk of a major stroke in the future. Patients should stop driving for at least 4 weeks after a TIA. Some referral units will want to use a scoring system, such as the $ABCD_2$ score (0–3 low risk, 4–5 moderate risk, 6–7 high risk) to determine the risk of the patient having a major stroke and how quickly the patient needs to be seen, so take measurements of all the parameters required to decipher the score:

- **A**ge ≥60 years – no: 0 points, yes: 1 point
- **B**lood pressure ≥140/90mmHg – no: 0 points, yes: 1 point
- **C**linical features – unilateral weakness: 2 points, speech disturbance without weakness: 1 point
- **D**uration of symptoms – ≤10 minutes: 0 points, 10–59 minutes: 1 point, ≥60 minutes: 2 points
- Known **D**iabetic – no: 0 points, yes: 1 point

14.6 Diplopia

14.6.1 Introduction

Diplopia occurs when the patient observes two of the same object. A number of conditions can cause this, but in primary care and A&E, when a patient presents saying *"I see two of everything"*, it is appropriate at the outset to determine if the patient sees double with both eyes open (binocular diplopia – which usually points to a neuro-ophthalmic or ocular misalignment cause) or with only one eye open (monocular diplopia – which usually points to an intraocular pathology such as refractive error or cataract).

A quick screening test to assess the type of diplopia the patient is experiencing, is to hold up an object (e.g. a pen) approximately 1 metre away and ask the patient to describe if they see one or two of that object. Repeat this when asking the patient to focus on a distant target such as a colleague working further away or a computer screen. Then ask the patient to cover each eye in turn, asking them to describe if they are still 'seeing two' with one eye covered. If the answer is 'yes', then this suggests a monocular diplopia rather than binocular diplopia. Monocular and binocular diplopia have different aetiologies and it is binocular diplopia where there is concern of a neurological pathology. The main cause of binocular diplopia is ocular misalignment or strabismus (see *Section 15.3.4*). Ocular causes of strabismus include orbital tumours, thyroid eye disease and orbital myopathy such as myasthenia gravis. The following are key associated features related to the ocular causes of strabismus:

- Orbital tumour
  - does the patient have globe displacement? (dystopia or proptosis, see *Chapter 7*)
  - does the patient have pain?
- Thyroid eye disease
  - does the patient have a previous diagnosis of thyroid dysfunction?
- Orbital myopathy
  - does the patient have variable ptosis, which is worse at the end of the day?
  - does the type of diplopia vary from day to day?
  - does the patient have breathing or swallowing problems, or choking episodes? (myasthenia gravis until proven otherwise).

The main non-ocular causes of strabismus are cranial nerve palsies (CNPs). Patients often have incomitant strabismus where measurements of the ocular deviation differ with direction of gaze.

14.6.2 Cranial nerve palsy

Table 14.1 illustrates the different cranial nerves involved in the movement of the eyes, namely CN III, IV and VI. As such, weaknesses in these nerves can lead to deficit in eye movement and abnormal eye position, which results in diplopia. The cranial nerves can be affected by:

- Microvascular conditions (cardiovascular risk factors)
- Macrovascular conditions
- Infective conditions
- Inflammatory conditions
- Neoplastic conditions.

CN III

The nucleus of CN III is in the midbrain at the level of the superior colliculus. It innervates the majority of the EOMs as well as the levator palpebrae superioris of the upper lid. Signs of cranial nerve palsy of CN III (CNP III) include:

- Ptosis
- Anisocoria (affected pupil larger than unaffected pupil and non-reactive/minimally reactive, especially in compressive CNP III)
- The eye in a down and out position (*Figure 14.3*).

Patients complain of horizontal and vertical diplopia (although this could be masked by the ptotic lid). Damage at its nucleus causes an ipsilateral CNP III with bilateral ptosis. Any damage caused to CN III in the path from its nucleus to the subarachnoid space can give rise to cranial nerve syndromes inclusive of ipsilateral CNP III, as follows:

- Nothnagel (contralateral hemiplegia)

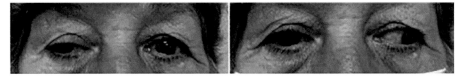

Figure 14.3 CN III palsy, with down and out position of right eye in primary position, and inability to adduct right eye, i.e. move right eye to the left.

- Benedikt (contralateral limb tremor)
- Weber's (contralateral limb hemiparesis).

During its course through the subarachnoid space, CN III runs lateral to the posterior communicating artery, causing pupil-involving CNP III. Ischaemic CNP III does not tend to involve the pupil; however, a new presentation of CNP III warrants urgent neuroimaging whether or not the pupil is involved (aneurysms of the posterior communicating artery are life-threatening and must be ruled out in the first instance).

CN IV

CN IV has its nucleus located in the midbrain, at the level of the inferior colliculus. It therefore has the longest intracranial course; it is often affected in closed head trauma.

As CN IV innervates the superior oblique, a CNP IV results in superior oblique underaction. The patient complains of vertical and torsional (tilted) double vision for distant and near objects. The affected eye is higher than the unaffected eye (i.e. hypertropia; *Figure 14.4*), with the height worse on contralateral gaze and ipsilateral head tilt (*Figure 14.5*).

Any damage at the nucleus, or along its path to the subarachnoid space, results in a contralateral CNP IV with RAPD, and ipsilateral Horner's syndrome and intention tremor. Within the subarachnoid space, the CN IV is most susceptible to trauma due to the long intracranial course (consider it as a possible cause in a patient with vertical diplopia after a head trauma).

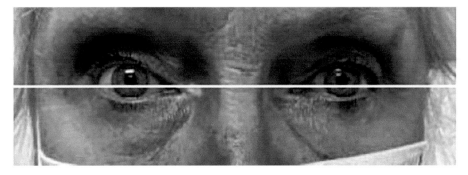

Figure 14.4 Hypertropia of the right eye in CNP IV (right eye at a higher position above the white line compared with the left eye).

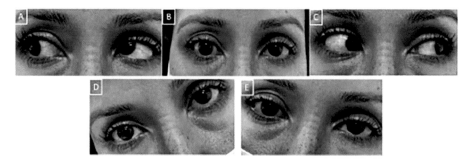

Figure 14.5 CN IV palsy, with hypertropia of the left eye (B), worse on right gaze (A) and left head tilt (E).

CN VI

The CN VI nucleus is located in the lower pons, anterior to the fourth ventricle and at the level of the facial colliculus. Damage at the level of the nucleus results in an ipsilateral CNP VI, with ipsilateral gaze palsy and palsy of CN VII. The patient complains of horizontal diplopia, worse at distance than near due to an inability to abduct the affected eye (*Figure 14.6*).

As the CN VI traverses to the subarachnoid space, damage to the fascicular portion of CN VI can cause the following syndromes as well as an ipsilateral CNP VI:

- Foville (ipsilateral horizontal gaze palsy, ipsilateral CNP VII, contralateral hemiparesis)
- Raymond (contralateral hemiparesis)
- Millard–Gubler (ipsilateral CNP VII).

Summary

A common cause for cranial nerve palsies, especially in a patient with cardiovascular risk factors (hypertension, diabetes and high cholesterol) is microvascular, but it is crucial to rule out GCA and neoplasm in any cranial nerve palsy cases, as well as more specifically:

- CN III palsy (eye down and out, ptosis): posterior communicating artery aneurysm
- CN IV palsy (vertical/torsional diplopia, head tilt): trauma
- CN VI palsy (horizontal diplopia): raised intracranial pressure causing a false localizing palsy.

Neuroimaging should also be considered if suspected 'microvascular' palsies do not resolve within the expected time frame (3–4 months).

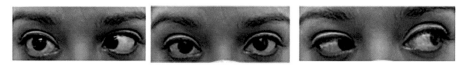

Figure 14.6 CN VI palsy with inability to abduct right eye (i.e. move right eye to the right).

Cavernous sinus syndrome

A patient presenting with multiple cranial nerve palsies including CN III, IV, V and VI, along with headache, proptosis and reduced vision, should raise a high suspicion for orbital pathology such as cavernous sinus syndrome. The most common cause of cavernous sinus syndrome is tumour, but cavernous sinus thrombosis should also be high on the list of differential diagnoses, particularly in the setting of dental infection or orbital cellulitis. This condition requires medical admission with urgent orbital imaging and venogram.

14.6.3 Management of diplopia

Diplopia warrants **urgent medical attention** if there are any red flag features (such as sudden onset, associated headache, loss of consciousness and seizure). These patients should be directed to their nearest emergency care centre where they can undergo emergency neuroimaging. If the cause of the diplopia is not clear, then **same day referral** to your local neuro-ophthalmology or ophthalmology department to assist with diagnosis is warranted.

Patients with diplopia should be followed up in a neuro-ophthalmology or strabismus clinic. In the acute setting, patching or stick-on Fresnel prisms can help alleviate the diplopia symptoms. In the long term, and once the underlying cause has been identified and treated (if appropriate) and there is stability in the ocular misalignment, prisms may be incorporated into the patient's glasses, or strabismus surgery may be performed to correct the ocular misalignment. Patients should be referred to the DVLA guidelines for advice on driving and informing agencies about diplopia.

14.7 Anisocoria

Anisocoria means unequal pupils. Assessment of the pupils must occur in bright and dim lighting conditions, so that it allows the clinician to assess the parasympathetic (involved in pupil constriction) and sympathetic (involved in pupil dilation) nervous systems.

Regardless of where the patient initially presents, history is important in determining what further investigations are warranted in anisocoria. Ask about:
- Onset
- Duration: *"when did someone tell you you had unequal pupils?"* or *"when did you first notice your pupils were unequal?"*
- Pain (*with neck pain think internal carotid artery dissecting aneurysm or apical tumour*).
- Associated neurological symptoms (*headache, diplopia, blurred vision, ptosis, limb weakness, paraesthesia*)
- Medication (*the caregiver who accidentally rubs their eyes after administering a hyoscine patch to a patient* – pharmacological anisocoria)
- Previous ocular surgery (*a complicated cataract surgery may lead to unequal pupil size*) or inflammation (*patient with recurrent episodes of uveitis*)
- Trauma (*blunt trauma can lead to iris sphincter tears and persistent dilated pupil*)
- Pain (*with neck pain think internal carotid artery dissecting aneurysm or apical tumour*).

A difference in diameter between the two pupils of ≤1mm in both bright and dim light with no ocular motility issue or ptosis is deemed physiological. Furthermore, if the pupils constrict to light, and briskly dilate to dark, there are no other abnormalities of the ocular examination and no other neurological symptoms, then it is also safe to say that any anisocoria of <1mm in both bright and dim light is also physiological. Pathological anisocoria is suspected when the amount of anisocoria is >1mm or differs between dim and bright lighting conditions.

Horner's syndrome presents with:
- Anisocoria (a pupil not dilating well in dim lighting, therefore appearing smaller (miosis) than the contralateral unaffected eye in dim light, but may be equal size in bright light)
- Partial ptosis
- Anhidrosis on affected side
- Heterochromia in congenital cases.

It is due to pathology (stroke, tumour, infection, trauma, demyelination) anywhere along the sympathetic chain (which extends from the hypothalamus, down through the brainstem and cervical cord, traverses the lung apex to ascend with the internal carotid artery through the cavernous sinus to reach the orbit), whether in the brain, neck or chest. Contrast this to a CNP III, where the pupil is fixed (or poorly reactive) and dilated, remaining the same in both bright and dim light, with a usually complete ptosis.

Pharmacological agents can be used in order to identify the location of the lesions causing the anisocoria. Apraclonidine 1% (Iopidine) can help diagnose a *presentation* of Horner's syndrome. When applied to the eyes of a patient with Horner's the affected eye will dilate, whereas in the unaffected eye it will not (reversal of the anisocoria). This test will not determine the *level* of pathology causing the Horner's syndrome (first order, such as stroke or demyelination; second order, such as neck dissection or Pancoast tumour; third order, such as internal carotid dissection or cavernous sinus thrombosis) and therefore all presentations of acquired Horner's syndrome need **urgent imaging: CT or MRI including angiography of the head and neck and thorax**. The *level* of the Horner's syndrome can further be determined with other pharmacological agents (see *Clinical Context tips* box below), but again, urgent imaging is still required regardless.

When there is more anisocoria in bright light conditions, and once a CNP III has been ruled out (eye is not in the down and out position and there is no limitation of ocular motility or ptosis), pupil constriction with pilocarpine 0.125% aids the diagnosis of a tonic pupil. If there is no constriction, pilocarpine 1% can be utilized; constriction with pilocarpine 1% suggests revisiting the diagnosis of a CNP III (*Section 14.6.2*).

How to pharmacologically determine the level of Horner's syndrome
Horner's syndrome is classified as central (from the hypothalamus to the ciliospinal centre of Budge), preganglionic (ciliospinal centre of Budge to the superior cervical ganglion) and postganglionic (from the superior cervical ganglion to the cavernous sinus). Although apraclonidine 1% facilitates the diagnosis of Horner's syndrome, to help isolate the level of the lesion the patient will need to be reviewed on a separate day using phenylephrine 1% – this causes dilation of the pupil in a postganglionic and not a preganglionic Horner's syndrome.

14.8 Visual field defects

Visual field defects are a result of pathology along the visual pathway. *Table 14.2* highlights some of the more common visual field defects and the part of the visual pathway that they correspond to.

Table 14.2 Visual field defects with symptom and pathology

Patient complaint	Visual field defect	Site of pathology
"I cannot see in the centre of my vision"		Macula Enlarged blind spot from optic nerve pathology
"I cannot see out of my left eye"		Optic nerve Total retinal detachment
"I cannot see my temporal field of view on either side"		Optic chiasm

Table 14.2 *cont'd*

Patient complaint	Visual field defect	Site of pathology
"I cannot see to my right side"		Optic tract
"I cannot see up and to the left"		Temporal optic radiation
"I cannot see down and to the left"		Parietal optic radiation
"I cannot see to my right side but my central vision seems OK"		Visual cortex / occipital lobe

Patients with VFD suggestive of optic chiasm or retrochiasmal disease require prompt neuroimaging. Depending on local hospital services, this could be expedited via a local A&E department, especially if stroke is suspected.

RED FLAG

Bilateral visual field defects are almost never bilateral retinal detachments. Any patient with bilateral loss of visual field of sudden onset has an intracranial pathology until proven otherwise, and requires urgent neuroimaging.

Chapter 15
Paediatric ophthalmology

15.1 Introduction

Children presenting to primary care or in the community can have a number of ocular complaints that can cause worry and anxiety to the patient, their carer(s) and, in some cases, other healthcare providers (particularly the midwife and health visitor).

The main sources of worry range from abnormal red reflex, to watery eyes, to the eyes spontaneously turning in or out. Here we will provide useful methods for examining children presenting with some of the most common paediatric ocular complaints, and discuss the best options for referral.

15.2 Paediatric history and examination

15.2.1 Paediatric history-taking

In *Section 1.1* a systematic approach to the history-taking of ophthalmology patients was discussed, focusing particularly on the presenting complaint and history of the presenting complaint. Gathering the history of a paediatric ophthalmology complaint follows a similar approach but additional information is required to ascertain when it is appropriate for the paediatric patient to be referred.

The following are quick reference points to questions that can be added to the general history-taking schema.

History
- Trauma with foreign objects or chemicals.

Carers' observations
- Eyes:
    - are the eyes red?
    - do the coloured parts of both eyes look the same or do either look cloudy?
- General or visual behaviour (particularly in preverbal children):
    - *"Do your child's eyes appear normal?"*
    - *"Is your child opening their eyes?"*
    - *"Is your child rubbing their eyes?"*
    - *"Does your child appear to dislike light?"*
    - *"Is your child holding the iPad close to their face or standing close to the television?"*
- **Associated symptoms:**
    - coryzal symptoms (current or recent)
    - nausea or vomiting
    - headaches
    - abnormal gait

   o changes in speech
   o systemic illness: fevers, reduced eating and drinking.

History-taking for any paediatric patient should also include:
- Birth history, including any perinatal infections of child or mother
- General health review
- Immunization history
- Developmental milestone history
- Family history of congenital eye disorders.

15.2.2 Examination of the paediatric patient

RED FLAG

There are some situations where examination is crucial and time-sensitive, for instance chemical ocular trauma where irrigation is imperative and sight-saving.

Examination of children can vary immensely and often depends on the comfort levels of the clinician, the cooperation of the child and, more importantly, the cooperation of their carer(s). The key is to make the environment as calming as possible for the patient, who is likely to be very scared and possibly in a lot of pain. Multiple attempts at examination by different members of the primary care or A&E team should not occur, because this will make subsequent examination by the ophthalmology team more difficult.

It can be helpful to observe the child's activity and behaviour in the waiting room. Are they refusing to open their eye(s)? Are they covering their eye(s) with their hand(s)? Do they seem to dislike light? Do they appear disorientated?

Once you have called the child into the consultation space, it is extremely important to build a rapport with them (and their carer(s)). Helpful tips include:
- Introduce yourself to the patient before their carer(s)
- In verbal children, ask them directly what is wrong, then ask them if you can ask their carer(s) some questions about them
- If they appear scared or upset, sometimes putting their favourite cartoon on your phone helps build trust
- Start by examining the child as soon as they come into the room (if you have a brief history taken at booking-in or triage), and *then* take a full, detailed history from the carer(s), to avoid the risk of the child losing interest (in adults of course, it is more common to take a full history first and then examine!)
- Start by describing what you are going to do as a game or lots of puzzles; their favourite cartoon or toy can help
- Offer to carry out the examination on either the patient's carer(s) or their favourite toy to show how easy it is (*Figure 15.1*).

The Brückner test, using the direct ophthalmoscope, and corneal light reflex test (Hirschberg test) with the same light source, address the following questions:

1. Is there an abnormality of the red reflex? (see *Section 15.3.1*; *Figure 15.2*)
2. Is there a refractive error?
3. Is there any ocular misalignment? (see *Section 15.3.4*; *Figure 15.3*).

In the Brückner test, the patient is seated comfortably, which could be in their carer's lap or their pushchair, in a dimly lit room (completely turn off the lights if possible). The direct ophthalmoscope should be set to 0. Look through the direct ophthalmoscope at a distance of approximately 60cm, ensuring the patient is fixating on the light of the ophthalmoscope. Both of the patient's eyes need to be illuminated simultaneously so that ocular alignment and symmetry of the red reflex can be evaluated. This test is invaluable in assessing for ocular pathology in a child.

The corneal light reflex test should be performed both binocularly and monocularly (*Figure 15.4*). For the monocular assessment, carer(s) can help occlude either eye. The behaviour of the patient with monocular occlusion can also give clues as to the vision in the unoccluded eye:

- If there is equal objection to occlusion, that suggests that vision is equal in both eyes
- If there is strong objection to occlusion of one eye, that would suggest the vision in the contralateral, unoccluded eye is suboptimal (*Figure 15.5*).

At the same time, assessing the corneal reflexes with monocular occlusion allows you to evaluate if the eye(s) remains central, steady and maintained (CSM, *Figure 15.4*).

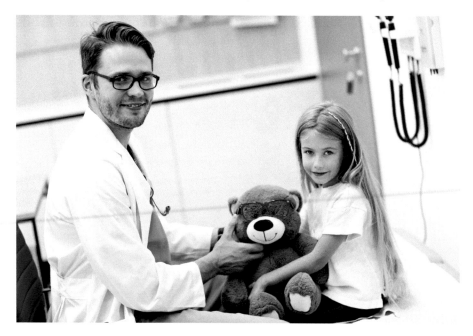

Figure 15.1 Clinician examining child's toy.

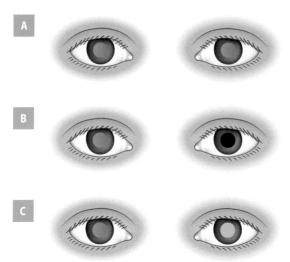

Figure 15.2 Abnormality of red reflex with Brückner test. (A) normal: child looks at light – both red reflections are equal; (B) unequal refraction – one red reflection is brighter than the other; (C) no reflex (cataract) – the presence of lens or other media opacities blocks the red reflection or diminishes it.

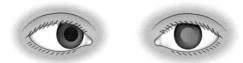

Figure 15.3 Ocular misalignment. In strabismus, the red reflection is more intense from the deviated eye.

Always consult your local policies on paediatric patient restraint, and always ensure that carer(s) are involved in the decision-making process.

Depending on the presenting complaint and if examination is too difficult, the patient will either be **referred for examination on a separate day** in the paediatric

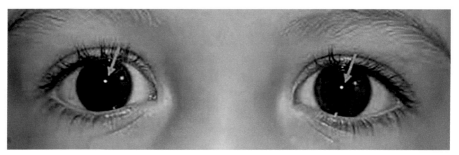

Figure 15.4 Corneal light reflex test (Hirschberg test).

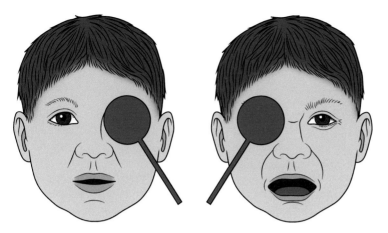

Figure 15.5 Monocular occlusion and the patient's reaction.

ophthalmology department or for examination under anaesthesia (for emergency cases). If examination under anaesthesia is required, consult early with the ophthalmology team and, importantly, note when the patient last had anything to eat and drink, and ensure that they are kept nil by mouth from that point forward. Ensure that this is communicated to the carer(s).

15.3 Common paediatric conditions

15.3.1 Abnormal red reflex

An abnormal red reflex can mean the red reflex is not as bright as may be expected, there is a clear difference in colour between each eye, or it is completely absent.

Causes
In children, the causes of abnormal red reflex can be broken down into the following subcategories:
1. Common causes: strabismus, refractive causes and racial differences
2. Life-threatening causes: retinoblastoma
3. Sight-threatening causes: corneal opacity, cataract and retinal detachment.

Investigation

In primary care or A&E you are not expected to dilate the patient to fully assess what the cause of the abnormal red reflex is, but you are expected to refer if you feel it is abnormal. *Section 15.2.2* describes briefly how to perform a Brückner test, which can provide information on the homogeneity and symmetry of the red reflex. *Figure 15.2* provides a reference guide for the types of abnormal red reflex that can be detected by the Brückner test with the direct ophthalmoscope. It is worth noting that a number of abnormal red reflex presentations can be caused by corneal pathology and, as such, initial examination of the cornea should be performed as described in *Section 2.5.2*.

Any paediatric patient with an abnormal red reflex will undergo a full anterior and posterior segment examination by the ophthalmology team, but the help of paediatric colleagues may be warranted for the full examination as well as full ocular motility examination and cycloplegic refraction.

Management

Abnormal red reflex requires **referral to a paediatric ophthalmologist**. The urgency of the referral is dependent on the history and initial clinical findings. For newborn patients, the national *Newborn and Infant Physical Examination* screening protocol (www.gov.uk/government/publications/newborn-and-infant-physical-examination-programme-handbook) dictates that any baby or infant with abnormal red reflex should be **reviewed by a paediatric ophthalmologist within 2 weeks**. A similar approach should be used for older children. Any suspicion of cancer should be **referred urgently for review within 1–2 weeks**.

Depending on the cause of the abnormal red reflex, the paediatric ophthalmology team will tailor management accordingly. For example, a newborn with congenital cataracts will need urgent surgery if the cataract is sufficiently affecting the visual axis.

15.3.2 Nasolacrimal duct obstruction

Nasolacrimal duct obstruction (NLDO) is observed in up to 20% of infants. NLDO occurs when the tear drainage system is not patent, and this inevitably causes a watery eye (epiphora), as well as crusting around the eyelashes secondary to dry mucoid discharge. Some children may have recurrent conjunctivitis as a result of NLDO and, in rare instances, a dacryocele, a bluish benign mass inferior to the medial canthus.

Causes

NLDO in children can be congenital or acquired (after coryzal symptoms or viral conjunctivitis) and is usually unilateral. Some syndromes with craniofacial abnormalities (for example, Down and Crouzon syndromes) have a higher incidence of NLDO due to anatomical variation of the bony structures that make up the nasolacrimal system.

Investigation

When a patient presents with a watery eye (*Figure 15.6*), the key question to ask the carer(s) is whether this started soon after they were born or whether it followed an episode of conjunctivitis. Carer(s) may also describe a mucoid discharge, with crusting of the eyelashes in the morning. Swabs are not usually necessary in these cases unless there is frank evidence of infection (conjunctivitis with a red eye; or dacryocystitis; see *Section 8.7*).

The ophthalmologist will assess the nasolacrimal system of the child in a number of ways. The initial assessment uses fluorescein 2% for the fluorescein disappearance test. One drop is instilled into each eye, and the time taken for the fluorescein to drain into the nasolacrimal system is recorded. The height of the tear lake, as illustrated in *Figure 15.6*, can also be recorded. The fluorescein will take longer to disappear from the affected side, and the tear lake will be higher.

RED FLAG

If a paediatric patient presents with persistent tearing / epiphora, photophobia and clouding of the cornea, congenital glaucoma must be ruled out.

Management

 Carer(s) can be reassured that most (around 95%) cases of congenital NLDO spontaneously resolve by 12 months of age. Until then, conservative measures include infant tear duct massage (also known as Crigler massage), whilst watching out for signs of infection (red / inflamed / sore eye) which may warrant topical antibiotic use. Mucoid discharge and crusting of the eyelashes can be removed by the carer(s) as necessary using cotton pads soaked in sterile water.

 If evidence of NLDO persists after the age of 12 months, or before this age if there are concerns of chronic conjunctivitis, dacryocele or dacryocystitis, patients should be referred to the paediatric ophthalmology service for further management. Surgical management involves syringe and probing of the nasolacrimal system to improve patency. In an older child, and where there is failure of syringe and probing and recurrent dacryocystitis, a dacryocystorhinostomy can be considered. Antibiotics have not been shown to be beneficial in non-infective NLDO.

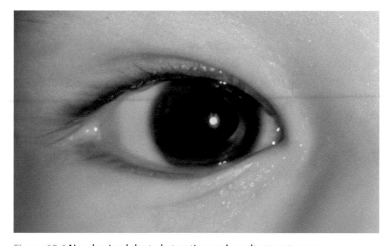

Figure 15.6 Nasolacrimal duct obstruction and resultant watery eye.

15.3.3 Neonatal conjunctivitis

Neonatal conjunctivitis, also known as ophthalmia neonatorum, is conjunctivitis that presents within the first 28 days of life. This should not be confused with NLDO. A patient with neonatal conjunctivitis presents with copious discharge and redness of the tarsal and bulbar conjunctiva, as well as evidence of preseptal cellulitis (*Figure 15.7*). The likelihood of neonatal conjunctivitis is dependent on the prenatal and perinatal history (particularly infections), as well as whether the patient was born by spontaneous vaginal delivery, caesarean section or with any intrapartum complications or infections. The most common pathogens involved in the aetiology of neonatal conjunctivitis can produce both sight-threatening and systemic complications, so it is imperative that the correct diagnosis is made.

Table 15.1 Common pathogens of neonatal conjunctivitis and timing of presentation

Timing of presentation	Likely pathogen
1–3 days	*Neisseria gonorrhoeae*
4–28 days	*Chlamydia trachomatis*
2–5 days	*Staphylococcus aureus*
	Streptococcus pneumoniae
	Streptococcus viridians
	Enterococcus spp.
	Haemophilus spp.
1–14 days	Herpes simplex

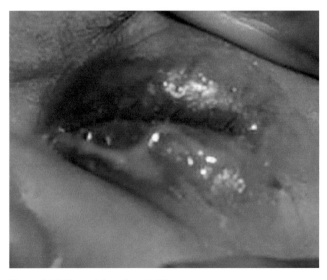

Figure 15.7 Neonatal conjunctivitis.

Causes

Table 15.1 shows the most common pathogens involved in the presentation of neonatal conjunctivitis (note that the list is not exhaustive). The speed of presentation, together with the history, can help determine the aetiology of the clinical presentation.

Investigations

Due to the clinical sequelae and complications of these pathogens, a strong clinical suspicion of neonatal conjunctivitis (conjunctivitis in a baby under 28 days of age), with the distinct clinical features highlighted above, warrants **same day referral** for specialist evaluation.

Specialists will take swabs for *Chlamydia trachomatis, Neisseria gonorrhoeae*, microscopy and sensitivity for bacterial infections, viral PCR and Gram stain, in these cases.

Management

Neonatal conjunctivitis patients need both topical and systemic treatment, and **same day referral** to the ophthalmology and paediatric teams at your local hospital is warranted to prevent life- or sight-threatening sequelae.

Topical treatment can be instigated by the ophthalmology team, but it is important that the patient is **referred to paediatric physicians for systemic treatment**, and further work-up as needed. These patients need close monitoring by the specialist MDT to ensure resolution, and to check that there are no complications of infection.

The diagnosis of neonatal conjunctivitis is particularly sensitive due to its relation to sexually transmitted infections. It is imperative to ensure that if any of the investigations are positive for sexually transmitted infections, that the carer(s) are referred to the local genito-urinary medicine clinic for appropriate treatment.

15.3.4 Strabismus

Strabismus, also known as ocular misalignment, describes any position of the eyes that deviate from the primary position. Children can present with cranial nerve palsies which cause incomitant ocular misalignment (see *Chapter 14*; ocular deviation does not measure the same in all directions of gaze), or they can have what is classed as comitant ocular deviation (ocular deviation measures the same in all directions of gaze).

Deviation of an eye should be evaluated by a paediatric ophthalmologist to ascertain the cause. This is with the caveat that there are no other neurological signs and symptoms, which if present means that **referral in the first instance should be to the paediatric medical team**, and before referral to the eye department.

Causes

Eye misalignment has both neurological and non-neurological causes. In children, amblyopia (failure in the development of the normal visual pathway with organic or non-organic causes) and refractive error are the most common causes of eye misalignment.

Investigations

 The first investigation that any clinician should do in a case of strabismus, whether as an acute or chronic presentation, is to ensure that extraocular muscle movements are full (see *Section 14.3*). If there is a limited range of eye movements, this may suggest a neurological problem and should be referred to the paediatric team. Eye movements can be assessed in small children with the assistance of their favourite toy, their carer(s) or their favourite cartoon on your phone (see *Figure 15.1*). Ask carer(s) to provide photographs so that you can check if the deviation was present previously.

RED FLAG

An acute esotropia in a paediatric patient with limitation of abduction would raise concern for an acute CN VI nerve palsy (see *Chapter 14*). This is a neurological emergency in this age group and requires referral to the paediatric neurology team for appropriate neuroimaging.

 The paediatric ophthalmology team will perform a full examination of the ductions (individual eye movements) and the versions (movement of both eyes in the same direction), to delineate if the strabismus has a neurological aetiology. A dilated fundoscopy to look for optic disc abnormalities and cycloplegic refraction would also be included in the ophthalmological work-up. Neuroimaging may also be required in certain circumstances.

Management

 In the primary care or A&E setting, a full history of onset of ocular misalignment and any associated signs and symptoms is imperative in delineating the time frame for referral, and governs the primary physician's treatment plan (Royal College of Ophthalmologists, 2012). Failure to refer to the correct team could lead to missed diagnoses. A multidisciplinary approach is needed to have the full clinical picture. A child with acute-onset strabismus and other neurological symptoms should be referred directly to the paediatric physician team who can then liaise with paediatric ophthalmology.

 Management by the ophthalmology team will be determined by the cause of the strabismus. It can vary from refractive correction, i.e. glasses to help keep the eyes straight, to patching to assist in the treatment of amblyopia, to neurological or neurosurgical input.

References and further reading

Pritchard, E., McAvoy, C.E. and McLoone, E. (2021) Rapid response to: Trust pays £7m for brain damage from failure to treat baby's eye infection. *BMJ*, **372:** n257.

Public Health England (2016, updated 2021) Newborn and Infant Physical Examination: programme handbook. Available at: www.gov.uk/government/publications/newborn-and-infant-physical-examination-programme-handbook

Royal College of Ophthalmologists (2012) *Guidelines for the Management of Strabismus in Childhood*. Available at: www.rcophth.ac.uk/wp-content/uploads/2021/08/2012-SCI-250-Guidelines-for-Management-of-Strabismus-in-Childhood-2012.pdf

Wong, R. *Tear Duct Massage (Crigler) for Infants* (video). Available at: www.youtube.com/watch?v=R-07jlKOg5U

Chapter 16
Trauma

16.1 Introduction

Ocular trauma can have serious consequences for the quality of life of a patient. Not only can the injuries be sight-threatening, but periorbital injuries also pose threats to cosmesis and function. The mechanism of trauma is important because it will provide clues as to whether there is an open or closed globe injury. The Birmingham Eye Trauma Terminology System (BETTS, *Figure 16.1*) covers both open and closed globe trauma and allows clinicians, whether in primary care, A&E or ophthalmology departments, to triage, manage and provide visual prognosis of ocular trauma.

This chapter provides a systematic approach to ocular trauma, guiding clinicians to best practice for their patients.

16.2 Trauma history and examination

16.2.1 History-taking

Section 1.1 provided a comprehensive review of the elements of history-taking of an ophthalmology patient. Most trauma cases allow history to be taken directly from the patient; however, In cases where the patient is unconscious, information on the mechanism of injury depends on collateral history. The following are key elements of any trauma history:

- Timing of injury
- Impact
- Mechanism

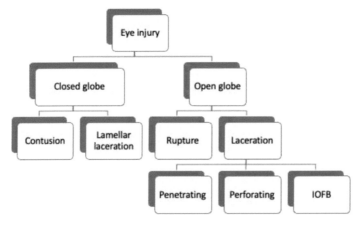

Figure 16.1 Birmingham Eye Trauma Terminology System. Adapted from Kuhn *et al.* (1996) A standardized classification of ocular trauma. *Ophthalmology*, **103**: 240, with permission from Elsevier.

- o high velocity
- o low velocity
- o chemical involvement
- Use of eye protection.

16.2.2 Examination

The most pertinent point to remember in suspected eye trauma is that minimal manipulation of the globe is extremely important. A heavy-handed approach could cause more trauma to an already compromised eye. *Figure 16.2* provides a useful reminder for any clinician who may encounter eye trauma in their practice.

If the globe is not readily visualized in the acute setting, an urgent CT of the orbits would be beneficial in ascertaining if the globe is intact. If eyelids are swollen shut due to ecchymosis, CT is extremely useful and will save excessive manipulation of the globe. If a CT is not readily available and the patient has already been referred to ophthalmology, a *gentle* ultrasound would also be beneficial in assessing the integrity

IF CHEMICAL INJURY, IMMEDIATE BEGIN IRRIGATING THE EYE

A — **Acuity** – visual acuity is the most important indicator of visual prognosis and should be checked first.

B — **Best** exam of **Both** eyes – the best exam begins with visual acuity. Using what's available (e.g. a penlight), examine both eyes from front to back. Ensure you don't apply any pressure to the globe during examination. Examine the uninjured eye first.

C — **Contiguous Structures. Contact Lenses** – assess all structures contiguous to the eye, including the eyelids, lacrimal drainage system, skin around the eye. As the eye is contiguous to the orbit and face assess the orbital rim and (if possible) for fractures. Note, but do not remove, contact lenses.

D — **Drugs, Diagnostics**, and "the **Don'ts**" – Administer IV or oral antibiotics with tetanus prophylaxis. Antiemetics and analgesics should be administered appropriately. Obtain a CT scan if possible. Don't apply pressure to the globe. Don't attempt ultrasound or get an MRI. Don't induce nausea/vomiting. Don't apply medications or dressings to the eye.

E — **Eye-Shield, Evacuate** – ensure an eye-shield is placed over the injured eye. Do not apply a dressing to the eye. Elevate the head if possible, and evacuate the patient to Ophthalmology urgently.

Figure 16.2 ABCDE of pre-ophthalmology ocular trauma care. Reproduced from Kroesen *et al.* (2020) ABCs of ocular trauma: adapting a familiar mnemonic for rapid eye examination in the pre ophthalmic zone of care. *Military Medicine*, **185**(Suppl 1): 448, with permission from Oxford University Press.

of the globe, but *only* if carried out by an experienced operator (see *Chapter 19* for more information on the use of ultrasonography).

RED FLAG

Trauma can have legal implications. You may be called upon to write reports at the request of the police if injuries are secondary to assault or non-accidental injury. Clear documentation is very important, and if there is concern about visual function, the patient should be referred to eye services the same day for baseline assessment.

16.2.3 How to make a globe trauma referral

 In cases of suspected globe rupture:
- Apply an eye shield to prevent extrusion of ocular contents
- Obtain or refer to A&E a CT orbits (see *Box 16.2*)
- Keep nil by mouth and start broad-spectrum IV antibiotics
- Emergency referral to ophthalmology.

When discussing a globe injury with your referral centre for ocular trauma, there are key questions that need answering on referral:

1. What was the mechanism of trauma?
2. Is the patient conscious or unconscious?
3. Has imaging been performed and what does it show?
4. Are you able to visualize any part of the globe?
5. Are the periocular structures intact (i.e. are there lid lacerations or degloving injuries)?
6. What is the vision of both eyes (with any glasses or contact lens the patient may wear)?
7. What are the pupillary reactions of both eyes? (is there a reverse RAPD, in other words, when you shine the pen torch on the compromised eye, does the opposite pupil dilate?)
8. Has tetanus status been checked?
9. When did the patient last have anything to eat or drink, and are they nil by mouth?
10. Are there any life-threatening injuries?

Remember life before sight. If the patient has life-threatening injuries, they will need stabilizing first before any ophthalmic surgery. Place a shield on the affected eye, and keep it in place until ophthalmology review.

16.3 Lid laceration

Chapter 2 described the anatomy of the eyelids. The eyelid limit is determined by the orbital rims. Traumatic lid lacerations can be simple or complex and caused by sharp or blunt trauma. The complexity of the repair depends on the involvement of the lid margin, involvement of the canalicular system, tissue loss, orbital fractures, and chemical or organic matter involvement. A generalized approach to the initial assessment of lid lacerations is as follows.

History of mechanism
- Road traffic collision, stab wound, animal bite
- Witnessed or unwitnessed (particularly for children).

Examination
- Full extent of laceration visualized
- Evidence of tissue loss or necrosis
- Nasolacrimal system involvement (medial canthal lacerations involve the canalicular system until proven otherwise)
- Evidence of globe injury.

Investigation
- If the globe is not visualized, low threshold for CT imaging.

Management
- Assess tetanus status (*Box 16.1*)
- Topical and systemic antibiotic cover for 'dirty' wounds (organic matter, animal bites)
- Surgical repair by ophthalmology.

BOX 16.1: ASSESSMENT OF TETANUS STATUS

- Is the ocular trauma classed as a tetanus-prone wound?
  - puncture wounds, wound with foreign bodies and animal bites and scratches acquired in a contaminated environment (i.e. soil-containing)
- Is your paediatric patient up to date with their vaccine schedule?
  - timepoints where children currently receive the tetanus vaccine: ages 8 weeks, 12 weeks, 16 weeks, 3 years and 14 years
- Has your adult patient had a tetanus vaccination within the last 10 years, as well as all childhood vaccinations?

When examining lid lacerations, minimal manipulation should occur if there is any concern regarding globe injury. Injuries involving the lid margin (*Figure 16.3A*) should assume a globe involvement unless proven otherwise. The globe should be visible (*Figure 16.3B*) and assessment of the eye continues as much as the patient will tolerate. If there is marked ecchymosis associated with the lid laceration which will not allow visualization of the globe, then CT imaging is warranted.

Without appropriate repair, the functional integrity and cosmesis of the eyelids is compromised. Superficial lacerations of the eyelid skin can be repaired in primary care or A&E using the appropriate absorbable suture (see below). Lid lacerations deeper

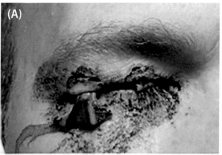
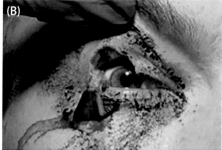

Figure 16.3 (A) Complex lid laceration with lid margin involvement; (B) visualization of the globe.

than the eyelid skin and involving the lid margin, canalicular system, orbital septum perforation and tarsal plate perforation, canthal tendons or tissue loss should **always be referred to ophthalmology or an oculoplastic service**. Most repairs should be performed within 48 hours to improve functional and cosmetic outcomes (although canalicular injuries should be sooner due to retraction, which can make repair technically difficult).

If referring to another hospital, covering the lid laceration with a damp sterile gauze will help with tissue viability. Think about keeping the patient nil by mouth (particularly children) in case general anaesthetic is required for repair that same day.

 Simple, small lid lacerations can be repaired in the ophthalmology treatment room, but more complex lacerations (nasolacrimal system involvement, orbital septum or fat prolapse, canthal tendon damage, involvement of the levator aponeurosis) should be repaired in theatre under general anaesthesia.

1. Position the patient in the supine position.
2. Obtain consent, explain the risks (infection, scarring, poor cosmesis, need for further surgical intervention) and benefits (prevent infection, retain function and improve cosmesis).
3. Apply topical anaesthetic eye drop to the surgical eye.
4. Assess the wound, documenting its extent and ensuring no deeper structures are involved. If the laceration is not complex, proceed with repair.
5. Inject subcutaneous local anaesthetic (e.g. 2% lidocaine with 1:100 000 adrenaline).
6. Clean the wound with sterile saline and assess further for any retained foreign body.
7. Avoid debriding any tissue if possible.
8. Absorbable sutures such as 6–0 or 7–0 Vicryl (polyglactin 910), are preferred (particularly for children) and are placed in an interrupted manner for skin and subcutaneous closure. A larger suture such as 5–0 Vicryl (polyglactin 910) is used for the tarsal plate and orbicularis closure.
9. Topical antibiotics should be prescribed (e.g. oc. chloramphenicol TID).
10. Any non-absorbable sutures used should be removed at clinic review in one week.

Lacerations involving the lid margin require careful closure to improve functional and cosmetic outcomes. The overriding principle is that the opposing sides of the laceration should meet and 'pout' to improve cosmesis and prevent notching of the lid. They should therefore only be repaired by your local ophthalmology or oculoplastic department.

16.4 Chemical injury

Chemical injury to the eyes can vary from mild to severe. Examples of the most dangerous alkaline substances are:
- Lime (found in plaster and cement)
- Ammonia (found in cleaning products and fertilizer)
- Lye (found in drain cleaner and airbags)
- Magnesium hydroxide (found in fireworks and sparklers).

Acidic agents that are particularly dangerous to the eyes are:
- Hydrofluoric acid (found in liquids used in the manufacture of herbicides, refrigerants and pharmaceuticals, as well as for the etching of glass)
- Sulphuric acid (found in bleach and refrigerants)
- Hydrochloric acid (found in swimming pools).

Alkaline substances are the most dangerous to the eye because their lipophilic nature allows them to penetrate tissues further, which makes their clearance more difficult. The only acidic substance that is able to cause as much damage as an alkaline substance is hydrofluoric acid, because it is able to penetrate the ocular tissues freely. This is in contrast to other acidic substances that denature proteins on contact, thereby preventing their penetration into the ocular tissues.

RED FLAG

Not all chemical injuries are caused by liquids. Powders can be just as dangerous and threatening to sight. Immediate treatment with copious irrigation still applies to such injuries.

Any patient presenting with a chemical injury to the eyes should undergo copious irrigation. Topical anaesthetic (tetracaine or proxymetacaine eye drops) should be administered to make irrigation more comfortable, but irrigation should not be withheld if this is not available. The patient should be positioned lying on their side so that the eye is irrigated with fluid flowing from the medial canthus to the lateral canthus (*Figure 16.4*). If available, a bag of normal saline with a giving set is useful for irrigation. The eyelids should be held open as much as possible (or a speculum placed) during irrigation to ensure the conjunctival fornices are also irrigated. **Immediate referral** to ophthalmology should be made to assess the extent of injury and instigate treatment. To make a referral to ophthalmology, the following are helpful points to remember for handover of the patient:

- Which chemical is involved?
- Are they medically cleared from an inhalation or ingestion point of view?
- One or both eyes involved? (always check the contralateral eye even if the history suggests only one eye was affected)
- Visual acuity
- Are the eyes red or 'marble white' (this can be assessed with a pen torch; a marble white eye suggests severe ocular burn and limbal ischaemia; *Figure 16.5*)
- Is the clarity of the iris equal on both sides? (a hazy cornea would suggest quite a significant burn)
- If fluorescein 2% is available, instil into the affected eye(s) and use a blue light to ascertain the extent of de-epithelialization (*Figure 16.6*).

 The following is a checklist for receiving a patient seen at either A&E or primary care with a chemical injury.

Immediate

- Assess pH: do not assume that the patient has been adequately irrigated prior to your assessment
- If pH remains >8 continue irrigation until the pH neutralizes (pH 7–7.5)
- If pH is neutral (7–7.5) inspect the adnexal and anterior segment structures:
  - evert the lids
  - inspect the fornices
  - assess for remaining chemical particulates (particularly with high pH chemicals such as cement and concrete); have a low threshold to continue irrigating.

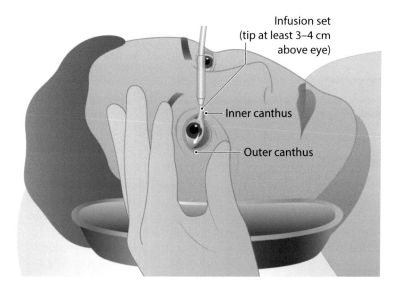

Figure 16.4 How to irrigate the eye. Adapted from Gwenhure, T. (202) Procedure for eye irrigation to treat ocular chemical injury. *Nursing Times*, **116(2):** 46, with permission.

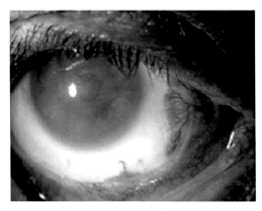

Figure 16.5 'Marbling' of conjunctiva suggestive of severe chemical injury. Reproduced from Dua, H.S. *et al.* (2020) Chemical eye injury: pathophysiology, assessment and management. *Eye*, **34:** 2001, with permission from Springer Nature.

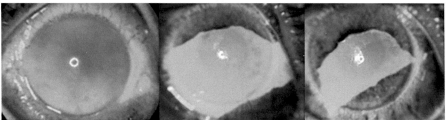

Figure 16.6 Varying levels of corneal and conjunctival de-epithelialization following a chemical injury, assessed with fluorescein sodium 2%. Reproduced from Dua, H.S. *et al.* (2020) Chemical eye injury: pathophysiology, assessment and management. *Eye*, **34:** 2001, with permission from Springer Nature.

Confirm the history

- Assess both eyes for evidence of chemical injury, even if the history suggests only one eye was affected
- Check IOP
- Assess the grade of injury:
  - instil fluorescein 2% into both eyes
  - the Roper-Hall and Dua classification (*Table 16.1*) allows for grading of ocular chemical injury – this is useful for documentation, monitoring progress and to provide a prognosis to the patient.

Treatment

- For all injuries think 'CLAAP':
  - **C**ycloplegic eye drops: to help with pain control and ciliary spasm
  - **L**ubricant eye drops: these must be administered regularly night and day (1–2-hourly depending on severity of burn)
  - **A**ntibiotic eye drops: this is to prevent infection, e.g. chloramphenicol 0.5% 4×/day
  - **A**nalgesia: simple analgesia such as paracetamol orally will help manage pain
  - All drops should preferably be **P**reservative-free

- Severe injuries (greater than Dua grade IV or Roper-Hall grade III):
  - consider admission if:
    - bilateral involvement
    - monocular patient
    - patient at risk of non-compliance (elderly, dementia)
  - CLAAP plus (CLAAP +):
    - topical steroids (preservative-free prednisolone 0.5–1% 4–6×/day depending on injury severity)
    - topical ascorbic acid 10% (preferred) or sodium citrate 10% (extremely irritant) every 2 hours
    - oral ascorbic acid (1g twice a day, but be careful in those with renal impairment)
    - tetracyclines can be considered because they help prevent tissue necrosis by inhibiting metalloproteinases (contraindicated in children under age 12, pregnancy and breastfeeding, renal and hepatic impairment)
    - amniotic membranes have also been shown to be useful due to their anti-inflammatory effects, but beneficial outcome only in mild and moderate burns compared to severe burns.

RED FLAG

The receiving ophthalmologist should always ask about ingestion or inhalation of chemicals. Laryngeal oedema, and subsequent deterioration, can be a late complication of both and the patient must be medically cleared by the A&E team, from an ingestion / poisoning point of view.

Table 16.1 The ocular surface burns classification systems of Roper-Hall and Dua

Roper-Hall classification of severity of ocular surface burns			
Grade	Corneal appearance	Limbal ischaemia	Prognosis
I	Clear cornea	Nil	Good
II	Hazy cornea: iris details visible	$<1/3$	Good
III	Opaque cornea: iris details obscured	$1/3$ to $1/2$	Guarded
IV	Opaque cornea: iris details obscured	$>1/2$	Poor

Dua classification of ocular surface burns			
Grade	Limbal involvement (clock hours)	Conjunctival involvement (%)	Prognosis
I	0	0	Very good
II	≤3	≤30	Good
III	>3–6	>30–50	Good
IV	>6–9	>50–75	Good to guarded
V	>9–12	>75–<100	Guarded to poor
VI	12 (total)	100 (total)	Very poor

Adapted from Roper-Hall, M.J. (1965) Thermal and chemical burns. *Trans Ophthalmol Soc UK*, **85:** 631 and Dua, H.S. *et al.* (2001) A new classification of ocular surface burns. *Br J Ophthalmol*, **85:** 1379.

16.5 Thermal injury

Thermal burns can be just as dangerous to the ocular structures as chemical injuries. In primary care and A&E, it is of utmost importance that the airway is stabilized and adequate fluid resuscitation is performed, due to the speed at which inhalation burns and laryngeal oedema can cause respiratory demise.

There are direct and indirect ways that thermal injuries can cause ocular surface damage, and so ophthalmology assessment is necessary. Treatment for ocular surface thermal injury is similar to that for chemical injury (CLAAP +), but for eyelids treatment is dependent on the thickness of burns. Full-thickness burns will often need surgical debridement, whilst superficial and partial burns need antibiotic prophylaxis as well as aggressive lubrication (lubricating ointment) in order to prevent cicatricial eyelid disease. There is a high risk of symblepharon formation, therefore regular ophthalmology assessment is necessary not only to surgically remove forniceal adhesions and pseudomembranes, but to assess for lagophthalmos (incomplete lid closure which can result in exposure keratopathy).

16.6 Orbital fractures

The most common orbital fracture secondary to blunt trauma is an orbital floor fracture ('blow-out fracture'). The orbital floor involves the zygomatic and maxillary facial bones (see *Section 2.2*) and is the weakest of all the orbital walls. *Table 16.2* illustrates some important symptoms and findings of an orbital floor fracture, and ways in which to assess them clinically in primary care, A&E and ophthalmology settings.

Table 16.2 Signs and symptoms of orbital fractures and how to assess them

Initial assessment	**Appropriate emergency resuscitation** (ABC)	
	History of mechanism of injury and symptoms	
	Examination: VA, pupils (particularly looking for RAPD), colour vision	
	Palpation of orbital rim to assess for discontinuity (see *Chapter 2* and *Figure 2.2*)	
	X-ray orbit (teardrop sign, *Figure 16.7*)	
	CT facial bones if X-ray is negative but clinical suspicion suggests orbital fracture (*Figure 16.8*)	
	Mechanism	**Assessment**
Periocular swelling	Ecchymosis Oedema Surgical emphysema	Palpate swelling ● Ecchymosis and oedema have a fluctuant feel ● Surgical emphysema (air in the subcutaneous tissue) – crackling or crepitus sensation on palpation
Malposition of the orbit	Extensive orbital fracture (mainly orbital floor)	Observe the patient for asymmetry of eye position or enophthalmos
Infraorbital paraesthesia	Orbital floor fractures traversing the infraorbital foramen or scar tissue compressing the nerve	Patient-reported numbness of the lower lid, ipsilateral nasal vestibule and upper lip Test with a wisp of cotton wool on both the affected and non-affected side for asymmetry
Diplopia	Muscle entrapment causing mechanical strabismus	Assessment of monocular or binocular diplopia (see *Section 14.6*)
Oculocardiac reflex	'Trapdoor' fractures in children Large orbital floor fractures in adults	Hypotension and bradycardia

Patients should be advised to avoid nose blowing, and can be placed on prophylactic broad-spectrum oral antibiotics on arrival. Orbital fractures are repaired surgically if there is evidence of entrapment, persistent symptomatic diplopia, over 50% of the orbital floor involved, or more emergently in the case of children – if there is cardiovascular compromise (oculocardiac reflex causing bradycardia). Refer to local guidelines as to whether ophthalmology or maxillofacial surgery repair these injuries, so that the appropriate referral can be made.

As noted in *Section 16.2.2*, there should be a low threshold for a CT scan if the globe cannot be fully visualized.

RED FLAG

A trauma patient with a tense orbit (tight eyelids, painful proptosis, reduced vision, RAPD, restricted eye movements) should be considered to have traumatic orbital compartment syndrome, which can cause irreversible sight loss, until proven otherwise. This is best treated with an emergency lateral canthotomy and cantholysis (see *Section 7.4.1* for a description of how to perform this procedure). It is important that it is performed by an experienced clinician. If there is any concern in primary care or A&E, then an urgent referral to the ophthalmology on-call service should be made.

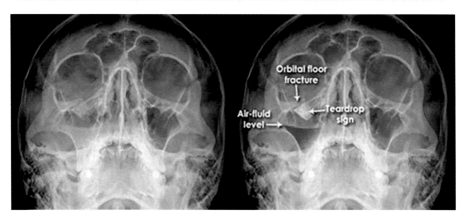

Figure 16.7 X-ray facial bones with right-sided teardrop sign and an air–fluid level indicative of a 'blow-out' fracture of the orbital floor. Reproduced from www.radiologymasterclass.co.uk with permission.

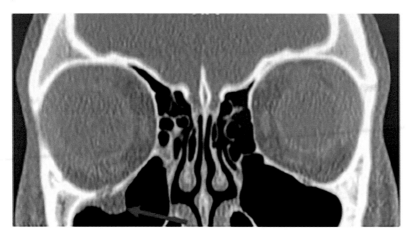

Figure 16.8 CT facial bones (coronal view) right-sided orbital floor fracture and inferior rectus entrapment (red arrow). Reproduced from Kumar, S., Artymowicz, A., Muscente, J. *et al.* (2023) Do not fall for this; diagnostic challenges in orbital floor fractures with extraocular muscle entrapment. *Cureus*, **15(2):** e35268, under a CC BY 4.0 licence.

16.7 Globe injuries

Globe injuries are classified as open or closed (see *Figure 16.1*). A variety of mechanisms can cause injury to the globe, and it is important to recognize that all ocular trauma should be referred urgently to your local ophthalmology service.

RED FLAG

A blunt trauma does not rule out a globe rupture.

16.7.1 Closed globe: contusion

A contusion, or bruise, can occur at both the anterior and posterior segments of the eye.

Subconjunctival haemorrhage (SCH) is a collection of blood under the conjunctiva of the eye. It can be spontaneous (consider after rubbing the eye in the patient on blood thinners, after a bout of coughing, or in a hypertensive patient) or as a direct trauma to the globe. Both blunt and sharp trauma can result in SCH; therefore, history is of utmost importance.

Isolated, spontaneous SCH does not warrant referral to your local eye services and will self-resolve over days to weeks. Anticoagulation does not need to be stopped. Any discomfort (most likely due to dellen formation) from bullous or raised SCH can be alleviated by frequent artificial tears. When a SCH is because of a trauma, **same day referral** to ophthalmology should be made to rule out open globe.

Hyphaema is the accumulation of blood between the cornea and the iris. It can range from microhyphaema (not visible to the naked eye or on assessment with a pen torch) to Grade IV, where the entire anterior chamber is filled with blood (*Figure 16.9*).

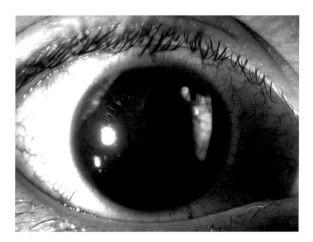

Figure 16.9 Hyphaema. Photo courtesy of Jacob Lang, OD, FAAO; previously published in: Lang, J. (2021) Hyphema. *Modern Optometry*, **3(5):** 76.

There should be a high index of suspicion of hyphaema in any ocular trauma. Whether spontaneous or secondary to trauma, visible hyphaema warrants **same day referral** to ophthalmology. In microhyphaema, and particularly with children, nausea, photophobia, blurred vision and headache may be presenting symptoms, and this also warrants **same day referral**.

A patient presenting with a history of ocular trauma from a primary care or A&E outside provider needs a comprehensive history and examination. Items to include in the initial assessment are:

History
- Date and time of injury
- Object that caused the injury
- Velocity of injury
- Eye protection
- Chemical involvement.

Examination
- VA
- IOP
- Pupils
- Visual fields to confrontation
- Anterior segment (use fluorescein 2% to assess continuity of cornea, conjunctiva and sclera)
- Gonioscopy (if tolerated)
- Dilated fundus examination
- CT scan to rule out globe rupture if suspected (see *Box 16.2*).

Management
- SCH
  - non-penetrating or perforating injury:
    - reassure
    - advise blood may take up to 14 days to resolve (more if the patient is on blood thinners)
    - advise use of artificial tears for ocular discomfort as a result of tear film disruption
  - penetrating or perforating injury:
    - treat as open globe injury (see *Section 16.7.4*)
- Hyphaema
  - absolute bed rest (consider admission for children who are unlikely to be compliant with eye drops or bed rest, or for high risk patients)
  - assess anticoagulant status (liaise with the medical team regarding withholding or reversal)
  - topical steroid 4×/day
  - topical cycloplegia (long-acting: cyclopentolate 1% twice daily or atropine 1% once daily)
  - daily review to assess IOP and ensure resolution

○ repeat gonioscopy at week 2 to assess for angle recession (3–6% risk of the development of glaucoma in these patients at 10 years, so regular follow-up is necessary).

RED FLAG

Remember that minimal manipulation of the globe is necessary when there is any suspicion of a globe rupture, as too much manipulation can cause expulsion of the eye contents through the open wound.

BOX 16.2: QUICK TIPS ON IMAGING FOR GLOBE INJURIES

Radiology request:
- Be very specific about injury and clinical findings
- Axial and coronal cuts, preferably 2mm slices, as well as soft tissue and bony windows should be requested.

Features on CT that help diagnose open globe injury include:
- Dislocated lens
- Intraocular haemorrhage
- Intraocular foreign body
- Intraocular gas
- Shallow or deep AC
- Globe deformity
- Wall irregularity.

16.7.2 Closed globe: posterior segment injury

The posterior segment can also be subject to non-perforating injury from blunt trauma. Injuries such as the following can all arise from blunt trauma:
- Commotio retinae (oedema of the retina, *Figure 16.10*)
- Choroidal rupture (sclera is intact but there has been a break in the RPE / Bruch's / choroid complex, see *Figure 16.10*)
- Traumatic optic neuropathy or optic nerve avulsion
- Retinal dialysis (full circumferential retinal break at the ora serrata)
- Traumatic macular holes.

These conditions can only be diagnosed after a dilated fundus examination. Aside from retinal dialysis and macular holes, there is no evidence-based treatment for these conditions, but they do pose a threat to visual function. A thorough baseline examination with ancillary testing as required will allow for monitoring of progression or recovery.

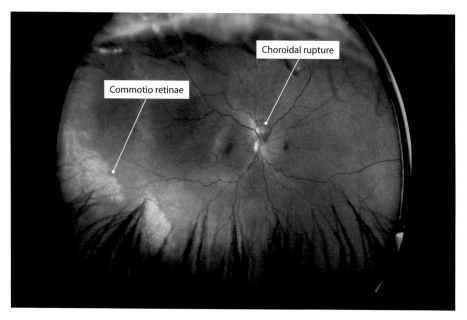

Figure 16.10 Commotio retinae and choroidal rupture (arrowed) in a patient after alleged assault.

16.7.3 Closed globe: lamellar laceration

A lamellar laceration is a *partial-thickness* corneal or scleral laceration. This is difficult to identify in primary care or A&E because assessment requires a slit lamp examination. The mechanism of injury provides clues, and it normally involves an injury with a sharp object (e.g. a piece of metal from welding, or a branch whilst gardening). History is important in this instance, and any ocular injury with a sharp object warrants **same day referral** to your local ophthalmology department.

In the ophthalmology setting, the systematic assessment of the ocular structures will follow a similar protocol to that described above (*Section 16.7.1*). Fluorescein 2%, topical anaesthesia and careful slit lamp examination is key in identifying aqueous leaks. In the case of lamellar lacerations, repair is warranted unless the wound has started to self-heal. Small, non-displaced corneal lamellar lacerations that have started to heal can be treated with topical antibiotics and a bandage contact lens, but generally corneal and scleral lamellar lacerations warrant surgical repair.

16.7.4 Open globe

An open globe injury is an ophthalmic emergency. Open globe injuries can be categorized into rupture and laceration, with laceration further subdivided into penetration, perforation and intraocular foreign body.

A rupture is caused by blunt trauma and breach of the continuity of the ocular shape at its weakest points (the limbus and just behind the insertion of the extraocular muscles). A penetrating open globe injury occurs when there is an entry wound, but no exit wound, and is caused by a high velocity or sharp object. A perforating open globe injury, on the other hand, describes where there is an entry and exit wound by the same mechanism.

Section 16.2.3 describes what should be undertaken in primary care and A&E when there is concern for an open globe injury, and how to make an appropriate referral to ophthalmology.

16.8 Non-accidental injury in children

Non-accidental injury (NAI) in children can involve marked trauma to both the eyes and orbital region. It is therefore imperative that documentation is precise, no matter whether the patient presents to A&E, primary care or ophthalmology.

Extensive periocular bruising and marked SCH in a child may warn of serious ocular trauma. In primary care and A&E the following assessments can all be performed: VA, visual fields (in older children), eye movement, assessing the bony orbit, appreciating any asymmetry in position of the globe, lids, conjunctiva, cornea, anterior chamber and pupils with a pen torch (see *Chapter 2*), as well as red reflex. Care must be taken not to excessively distress the paediatric patient, particularly in cases of suspected globe rupture, and minimal manipulation of the orbit and globe should occur. Prompt analgesia is beneficial in children and can facilitate careful examination (see *Section 15.2.2* for tips on how to examine a child).

Ophthalmologists are often called upon to perform dilated fundoscopy to exclude retinal haemorrhages in cases of NAI. However, it is important for ophthalmologists to also recognize non-ophthalmic features of physical abuse which may prompt referral to the paediatric team and the named consultant for NAI. **It is important to know your local guidelines regarding protocols in place for making an NAI referral.** *Table 16.3* includes a quick reference guide for ophthalmologists regarding what to look out for and what to do in cases of suspected NAI (for more information review the RCOphth and RCPCH guideline *Abusive Head Trauma and the Eye in Infancy*: www. rcophth.ac.uk/wp-content/uploads/2021/08/2013-SCI-292-ABUSIVE-HEAD-TRAUMA-AND-THE-EYE-FINAL-at-June-2013.pdf)

Table 16.3 Quick reference guide for ophthalmologists to management of non-accidental injury cases

Findings	What to do	Documentation
Ophthalmic ● Periocular bruising and lacerations ● Unexplained lens dislocation or cataract ● Unexplained conjunctival or corneal injuries (lower half of the eye) ● Retinal haemorrhages **Non-ophthalmic** ● Bite marks ● Bruising in non-mobile infants ● Contact burns on face and hands	1. Trainees should discuss with the consultant on call or the paediatric ophthalmology team 2. Suspicion of NAI should be confirmed by a senior 3. Referral should be made to the safeguarding team 4. Referral to be communicated to the family including your concerns and reasons for referral	1. Date and time of encounter 2. Name and grade 3. Name and grade of referring team 4. History (information regarding the environment and factors surrounding the injury are key and must be clearly documented) 5. Findings (see *Figure 16.11* for the RCOphth proforma for documenting ophthalmic findings in NAI and abusive head trauma)

References and further reading

Clare, G., Bunce, C. and Tuft, S. (2022) Amniotic membrane transplantation for acute ocular burns. *Cochrane Database Syst Rev*, **9(9):** CD009379.

Public Health England (2019) *Management of Tetanus Prone Wounds*. Available at: https://assets.publishing.service.gov.uk/government/uploads/system/uploads/attachment_data/file/849464/Tetanus_tetanus_prone_injury_poster.pdf

Public Health England (2019) *Post Exposure Management for Tetanus Prone Wounds*. Available at: https://assets.publishing.service.gov.uk/government/uploads/system/uploads/attachment_data/file/849460/Tetanus_quick_guide_poster.pdf

RECORDING OF OPHTHAMOLOGICAL FEATURES
IN SUSPECTED PAEDIATRIC HEAD TRAUMA

HISTORY
Continue on reverse

PATIENTS DETAILS

If possible to assess

Visual Acuity	Right eye	Left eye

OCULAR MOTILITY

Right eye   Left eye

Pupil size and Pupillary reflexes	**PERIOCULAR BRUISING:** (mark areas of bruising)

SUBCONJUNCTIVAL HAEMORRHAGES

Right eye		Left eye	
Yes	No	Yes	No

Pupils dilated with	

ANTERIOR SEGMENT

Right Eye	Left Eye

Circle single or multiple appropriate responses if present or enter free text

FUNDUS Circle if present	RIGHT EYE				LEFT EYE			
Retinal Haemorrhages	YES		NO		YES		NO	
NUMBER of Retinal haemorrhage	Few (1-10)	Many(10-20)	Too numerous to count		Few (1-10)	Many(10-20)	Too numerous to count	
LOCATION of retinal haemorrhages	Pre retinal	Intraretinal	Subretinal	Multilayered	Pre retinal	Intraretinal	Subretinal	Multilayered
DISTRIBUTION of retinal haemorrhages	Posterior Pole Few/many/ too numerous to count (Zone 1: ROP classification)		Periphery Few/many/ too numerous to count (outside Zone 1)		Posterior Pole Few/many/ too numerous to count (Zone 1: ROP classification)		Periphery Few/many/ too numerous to count (outside Zone 1)	
SIZE of retinal haemorrhages	Small (< 1dd)	Medium 1-2dd	Large >2dd		Small (< 1dd)	Medium 1-2dd	Large >2dd	
MORPHOLOGY of haemorrhages White centered or other								
Macula Retinoschisis								
Perimacular folds								
Optic disc								
OTHER findings								

Name and signature	
Date and time of examination	

Fundus examined with
Indirect ophthalmoscope (and 20d / 28d / 30d / 2.2d)

Retcam	OR Photography
OCT	

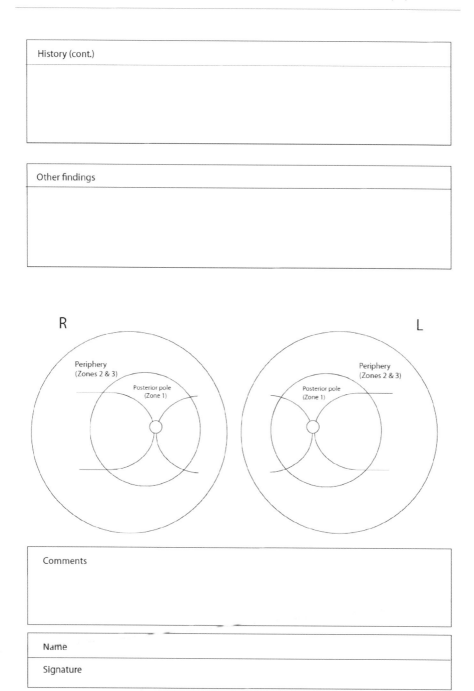

History (cont.)

Other findings

R

L

Periphery
(Zones 2 & 3)

Posterior pole
(Zone 1)

Periphery
(Zones 2 & 3)

Posterior pole
(Zone 1)

Comments

Name

Signature

Figure 16.11 Royal College of Ophthalmologists proforma for recording ophthalmological features in suspected paediatric head trauma. Reproduced from www.rcophth.ac.uk/wp-content/uploads/2021/08/2013-SCI-292-ABUSIVE-HEAD-TRAUMA-AND-THE-EYE-FINAL-at-June-2013.pdf with permission.

Chapter 17
Visual fields

17.1 What is a visual field test and why do we use it?

The visual field test (also known as perimetry) is a measure of the area seen when the patient's gaze is fixed on a central target. This is an investigation you will come across in the glaucoma clinic, but it is also used to evaluate and follow the progression of any optic neuropathy. The importance of the visual field test in glaucoma cannot be overstated, because losses can be picked up earlier by the test than the patient themselves reporting symptoms. In glaucoma visual field damage is irreversible, so good interpretation of this test for early diagnosis, monitoring and prevention is vital.

Visual fields is also a very useful test for other disorders, such as localizing and monitoring the visual function effects of intracranial lesions and certain retinopathies (e.g. hydroxychloroquine retinopathy), and also for patients presenting with vague visual complaints who have no apparent discernible pathology on clinical examination.

17.2 The visual field

The visual field extends 50° superiorly, 60° nasally, 70° inferiorly, and 90° temporally. The field is sharpest at the fovea and then declines in the periphery, with the nasal slope steeper than the temporal. The physiological blind spot is located temporally between 10° and 20°, slightly below the horizontal meridian.

17.3 Types of visual field test

Visual fields can be tested in either of the following manners:
- **Kinetic**: where the target moves from a non-seeing to a seeing area, and the point at which the target is first seen is documented; e.g. Goldmann perimetry test
- **Static** (most types of automated perimetry): where the stimulus is stationary (at pre-selected locations in the visual field) but changes in intensity until the sensitivity (or threshold) of the eye at that point is found; e.g. Humphrey visual field.

17.4 Common terms in visual field testing

- **Scotoma**: an area of visual loss (either absolute or relative), surrounded by a seeing area
- **Isopter**: a threshold line that joins points of equal sensitivity on a visual field chart, enclosing an area within which a stimulus of a given strength is visible
- **Homonymous**: the defects are in corresponding areas of visual fields in both eyes (see *Section 14.8*)
- **Congruous**: how 'matched' the defect is, i.e. how similar the defect is between the eyes. Usually, the more matched, the more posterior the lesion.

17.5 Interpreting visual field tests

Humphrey perimetry testing is the most clinically utilized visual field test in the UK. The methodology below is based on this test, though the principles can be used to interpret most visual field tests.

The most commonly used Humphrey protocol is '24–2', meaning the central 24° from fixation is tested (i.e. 48° altogether).

17.5.1 Positioning

Ensure the patient's left eye print-out is on the left side of the page and the right eye print-out is on the right side of the page (see *Figure 17.1* for a normal result). The field should read as if *you* are the patient! This is the opposite to most eye investigation / examination reports, which are usually laid out as if you are *looking at* the patient (i.e. patient's right on your left, patient's left on your right).

17.5.2 Basics

Confirm the patient demographics, and time and date of the test.

17.5.3 Testing strategy

Check the test strategy used, the stimulus size, intensity and background luminance details. These should be consistent when compared to the patient's last test.

17.5.4 Reliability indices

1. Fixation losses: indicating patient eye movements, i.e. the patient responding when a target is presented into the mapped physiological blind spot, or via pupil tracking.
2. False positives: the patient responding when there is no stimulus ('trigger happy').
3. False negatives: the patient fails to respond to a suprathreshold stimulus at a location that was previously responded to (e.g. if malingering, tired).

The time taken to complete the test can also give an indication as to its reliability (i.e. an extremely slow or extremely fast test may be less reliable).

17.5.5 Sensitivity and summary values

1. Numerical display: a numerical representation of the field. The larger the number, the more the light was attenuated, i.e. the dimmer the target that was seen.
2. Greyscale: a graphical representation of the numerical display, with darker points indicating decreased sensitivity.
3. Total deviation: compares the patient to age-matched controls.
4. GHT ('glaucoma hemifield test'): this compares five points on the upper part of the field to five corresponding points on the lower part of the field. This allows assessment of visual field damage in patterns that are commonly seen in glaucoma (*Figure 17.2*).
5. VFI ('visual field index'): this quantifies the visual field as a percentage of field function by age (where 100 is normal, and greater weight is given to points closer to fixation).

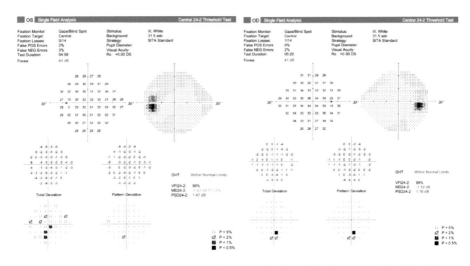

Figure 17.1 Humphrey perimetry test (normal test result). The left field is on the left side of the page and the right field is on the right side of the page (as if you are the patient). The patient demographics and date of test are not shown here, but should be checked. The strategy used is SITA standard (Swedish Interactive Thresholding Algorithm – the machine's method for testing). The reliability indices show a relatively reliable test, with low fixation losses, false positives and false negatives in both eyes. The greyscale shows physiological blind spots in the temporal fields of both eyes. Though there are some scanty losses of sensitivity shown on the total deviation, the pattern deviation has corrected for generalized depression and indicates a field within normal limits.

6. Mean deviation: averages the departure of each test point from age-adjusted values (poorer results indicated by more negative values).
7. Pattern standard deviation: adjusts for generalized depressions in the overall field (highlighting focal depressions, which may otherwise be masked by, for instance, media opacity; poorer results indicated by more positive values).

CLINICAL CONTEXT TIPS

Ensure that you have the correct patient and that the field is reliable. Ask yourself if the field is within normal limits. If not, is it one eye (indicating the damage is in front of the optic chiasm) or both eyes (either separate damage anterior to the chiasm, or damage to the chiasm/post-chiasmal)? Where is the region and shape of the defect? Don't forget to compare to the patient's previous field(s).

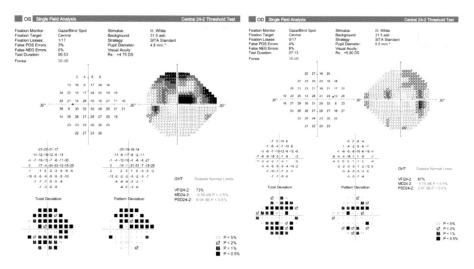

Figure 17.2 Humphrey perimetry test (glaucomatous field changes). The left field is on the left side of the page and the right field is on the right side of the page, as if you are the patient. The patient demographics and date of test are not shown here, but should be checked. The strategy used is SITA standard. The reliability indices show a relatively reliable test in the left eye though slightly less so in the right eye, with higher false positives and false negatives. The greyscale shows a superior arcuate defect and a paracentral scotoma in the left eye, and start of a superior arcuate and paracentral defect in the right eye; both coming through on pattern deviation. The glaucoma hemifield test is also outside normal limits.

CLINICAL CONTEXT TIPS

What can affect field results?

- Poor performance
- Uncorrected refractive error
- Spectacles
- Ptosis
- Miosis / mydriasis
- Media opacities
- Inadequate retinal adaptation (e.g. following slit lamp examination)
- Technical skill of perimetrist.

Chapter 18

Ocular coherence tomography

18.1 What is ocular coherence tomography and why do we use it?

Ocular coherence tomography, or OCT, is a non-invasive imaging modality commonly used in the eye clinic, which allows cross-sectional analysis of both the anterior and posterior segments.

18.1.1 How does it work?

OCT uses the principles of light interferometry, using light in the infrared spectrum (810nm). A partially reflective mirror is used to split the coherent (incoming) light into a measuring beam (which is directed into the eye, where different tissues reflect the beam to differing extents) and a reference beam (which is directed to a reference mirror).

Images are created by analysing the resulting interference, i.e. interaction between the reflected reference waves and the waves reflected by the ocular tissues.

As OCT relies on light, conditions which cause media opacity, such as corneal opacity, dense cataract and vitreous haemorrhage, can impede the progress of light and hence affect the image quality. Patient cooperation is also required, as the ability to fix on a target during the test is required.

18.2 What types of OCT are there?

OCT can be used for different parts of the eye:
- Anterior segment: for detailed views of the cornea, anterior chamber and visualizing the iridocorneal angle
- Retinal nerve fibre layer: a circular OCT scan centred on the optic nerve head; often used in glaucoma clinic as a visual quantitative inspection of retinal ganglion cell axonal loss (and therefore glaucomatous damage), compared to age-matched controls
- Optic nerve: useful for visualizing optic nerve drusen or swelling
- Macula: mainstay of diagnosis and progression-monitoring for most medical retina conditions; macular OCT can also be useful in clinical assessment of patients with loss of vision with subtle pathology, where clinical examination does not reveal overt findings.

The following is mainly a discussion of macular OCT.

18.3 Macular OCT

18.3.1 Retinal anatomy

To understand macular OCT, it is vital to have a good grasp of retinal anatomy (see *Section 2.9* for full details and *Figure 18.1* for the corresponding OCT).

18.3.2 A normal macular OCT

OCT images the retinal layers in cross-section. To better understand this, imagine the retina as an iced cake. When we look at the retina on the slit lamp, we are looking at the retina from the top, i.e. holding the cake up in front of us on its side, looking at the top icing (with all the posterior layers hidden behind it). When we are looking at the OCT of the macula, imagine we are putting the cake on the table, slicing it in half and looking side-on at each of the layers. The top of the image you are looking at is the inner retina, the bottom is the outer retina and choroid.

On an OCT, the different layers exhibit differing extents of reflectivity:
- Inner limiting membrane (ILM): not visibly depicted on an OCT
- Nerve fibre layer (NFL): hyperreflective
- Ganglion cell layer (GCL): hyporeflective
- Inner plexiform layer (IPL): hyperreflective
- Inner nuclear layer (INL): hyporeflective
- Outer plexiform layer (OPL): hyperreflective
- Outer nuclear layer (ONL): hyporeflective
- External limiting membrane (ELM): hyperreflective
- Photoreceptor layer – ellipsoid zone (PL-EZ) and interdigitation zone (PL-IZ): hyperreflective
- Retinal pigment epithelium (RPE): three hyperreflective bands.

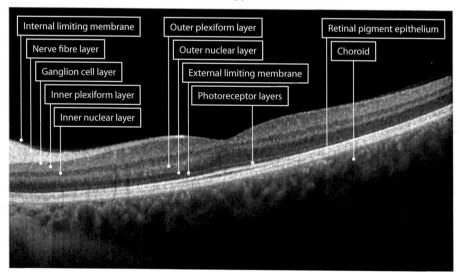

Figure 18.1 Retinal topography and cross-section.

Figure 18.2 shows a normal, healthy macular OCT. You can identify which eye this is an OCT of, as with the image on the left a part of the optic nerve is seen to the right, and with the image on the right, the nerve fibre layer is thickest to the right of the image; both illustrating this is the right eye. The dip in the centre, shown in the image on the right, is the fovea. If this normal 'dip' contour is lost, it can be due either to outer retinal pathology (e.g. macular oedema) or vitreoretinal anomalies (such as vitreomacular traction or epiretinal membranes). The premacular vitreous and choroid can also be visualized. The clivus is the curved walls either side of the fovea.

18.3.3 Interpreting macular OCT

1. Check patient demographics and date and time of the test, especially when the same patient has had multiple scans over a long period of time.
2. Check the signal quality (often documented as a number out of ten); the higher the number, the better the scan quality. Ensure the scan is centred on the fovea; note that this may not be possible for patients with very poor vision who cannot fixate on a small target.
3. Compare left and right eye scans simultaneously to ensure that you do not forget to review one eye's scan.
4. Note any positive findings and relevant negative findings (see next section).
5. Compare to the patient's previous scans.

18.3.4 Macular OCT findings

Hyporeflective (dark) areas
On a macular OCT these usually represent fluid. This fluid can be intraretinal (*Figures 18.3–18.5*), sub-retinal or sub-RPE (*Figure 18.6*). Causes of cystoid macular oedema are shown in *Box 18.1*.

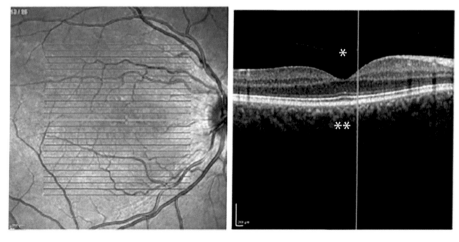

Figure 18.2 Normal macular OCT. Left: infrared image. Right: cross-section through the highlighted green line. One white star: premacular vitreous; two white stars: choroid.

Hyperreflective (light / white) areas

On a macular OCT these could represent hard exudates (*Figure 18.7*), drusen (*Figure 18.8*), haemorrhages, fibrosis (*Figure 18.9*), membranes (e.g. choroidal neovascularization) or vitreous opacities.

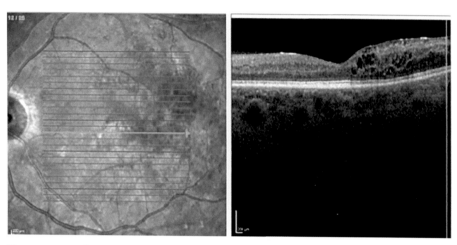

Figure 18.3 Focal cystic pockets of intraretinal fluid just temporal to the fovea in diabetic macular oedema (left eye).

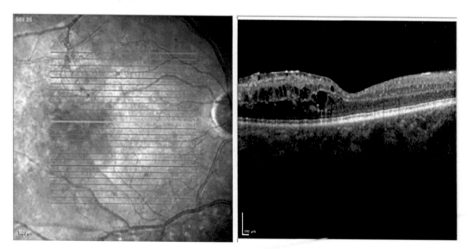

Figure 18.4 Focal area of larger intraretinal cysts just temporal to the fovea in diabetic macular oedema (right eye).

223

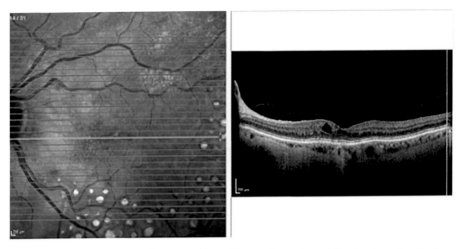

Figure 18.5 Solitary intraretinal cyst in patient with macular oedema following branch retinal vein occlusion. The circular scars seen at the inferior macula on the infrared image on the left are from sectoral panretinal photocoagulation (left eye).

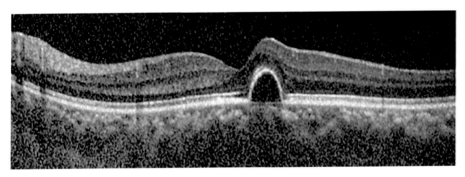

Figure 18.6 Focal hyporeflective area sub-retinal pigment epithelium (RPE), i.e. a serous pigment epithelial detachment in choroidal neovascularization (left eye). In contrast, fluid above the 'bright white line' of the RPE would be termed sub-retinal fluid.

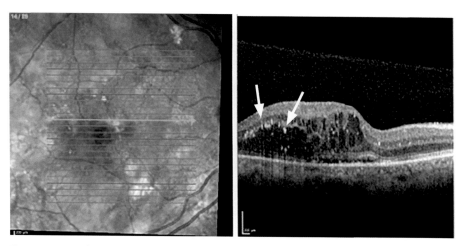

Figure 18.7 In addition to the temporal intraretinal fluid seen, multiple hyperreflective dots (white arrow) are visible which are exudates in a patient with a retinal vein occlusion with macular oedema (right eye).

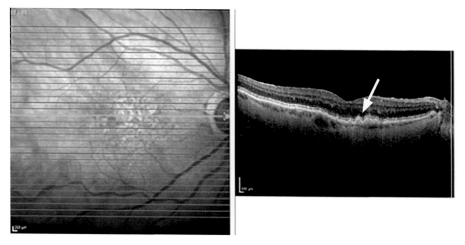

Figure 18.8 The homogeneous hyperreflective areas under the undulating retinal pigment epithelium represent drusenoid pigment epithelial detachment (white arrow) causing disruption of the ellipsoid zone in this patient with dry age-related macular degeneration (right eye).

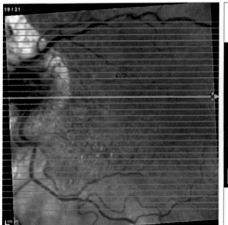
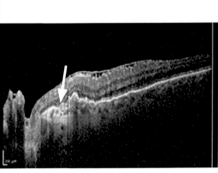

Figure 18.9 The heterogeneous hyperreflective areas under the undulating retinal pigment epithelium represent fibrovascular pigment epithelial detachments (white arrow) in this patient with wet age-related macular degeneration. The thin hyperreflective membrane seen overlying the macula is an epiretinal membrane (left eye).

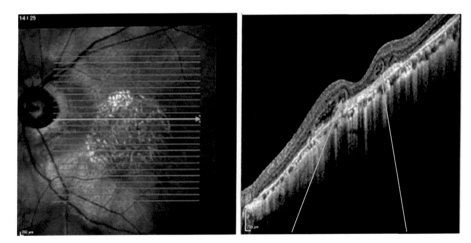

Figure 18.10 The obvious hyperreflective area here represents central scarring and fibrosis in this patient with poor vision from myopic choroidal neovascularization. However, looking closely you will also see two hyporeflective 'rings' surrounded by hyperreflective rims (arrowed). These are outer retinal tubulations in the outer nuclear layer and are a sign of end-stage retinal degeneration. It is vital to differentiate these from intraretinal cysts (which would be a sign of angiogenic activity and may spur a clinician to continue intravitreal injections).

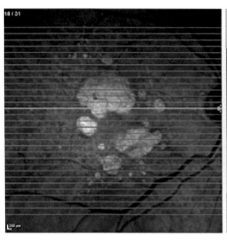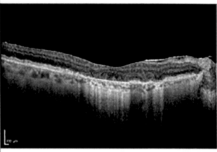

Figure 18.11 Atrophy – loss of outer retinal layers (also resulting in increased choroidal hyperreflectivity over the areas where the retina is thinned and the OCT signal penetrates further). Disruption of these layers is causing this patient with end-stage age-related macular degeneration to have poor vision (right eye).

CLINICAL CONTEXT TIPS

The **inner** retina (towards the top of the OCT image) is affected by retinal vascular disease. In chronic ischaemia, the inner layers will appear thinned and atrophic. In acute retinal artery obstruction, the inner layers will initially appear thickened and more hyperreflective.

The **outer** retina (towards the bottom of the OCT image) is affected by inflammation, retinal vascular and choroidal vascular disease. Fluid here can be related to the many causes of macular oedema.

BOX 18.1: CAUSES OF CYSTOID MACULAR OEDEMA

- Vascular disease: retinal vein occlusion, diabetic retinopathy
- Degenerative disease: choroidal neovascularization, e.g. wet age-related macular degeneration
- Inflammatory: post-operative, posterior uveitis
- Drug-related: topical prostaglandin analogues
- Inherited: retinitis pigmentosa
- Traction-related: vitreomacular traction, epiretinal membrane causing a 'pulling' effect with cystoid macular spaces
- Tumours of the posterior segment
- Optic disc anomalies, e.g. optic disc pit.

Chapter 19
Ocular ultrasound

19.1 What is an ocular ultrasound and why do we use it?

To understand ocular ultrasound, it is important to understand the key principles of ultrasound. Ultrasound scanning is a generally safe, low cost imaging modality which does not use ionizing radiation and gives valuable real-time information to the clinician.

Ultrasound uses a principle called acoustic impedance, which is a measure of a medium's resistance to sound passing through it; it is defined as its density multiplied by the sound velocity. A piezoelectric crystal within the probe is electrically stimulated to vibrate and emit high frequency sound waves of 8–10MHz into the eye. When a sound wave strikes an interface between structures of differing acoustic impedance, part of the wave is reflected back to the transducer as an echo. This energy re-stimulates the crystal, and its mechanical vibrations are converted to an electric current, which is displayed on the visual screen as dots or lines.

The two main types of ocular ultrasound are A scan and B scan. A and B scans can be performed simultaneously on one patient. An A scan (amplitude mode) probe creates a parallel 8MHz sound beam, resulting in an image composed of spikes of varying heights along a baseline (*Figure 19.1*). A scans are useful for measuring the eye's axial length, differentiating intraocular membranes, or identifying intraocular lesions. B scan is more commonly used to assess pathology in clinic (*Figure 19.2*).

A B scan (brightness mode) probe's oscillating crystal creates focused 10–15MHz sound waves, resulting in an image composed of dots of varying brightness. B scans are useful in documenting the contours and topographic arrangement of intraocular structures.

Anterior segment ultrasound (ultrasound biomicroscopy or UBM), is a B scan utilizing higher frequencies of 50–100MHz to image the anterior parts of the eye, such as the cornea, iris and lens. Though these images have better resolution, the shorter wavelengths produce a signal with insufficient depth of penetration to reach the posterior structures within the eye.

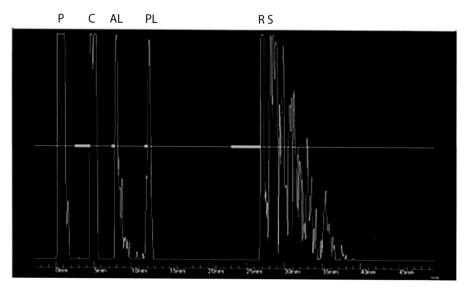

Figure 19.1 A scan showing normal spikes. From left to right the spikes represent: the probe (P), the cornea (C), the anterior lens (AL), the posterior lens (PL), the retina (R) and the sclera (S). The collection of spikes at the right of the image represents the orbital tissues.

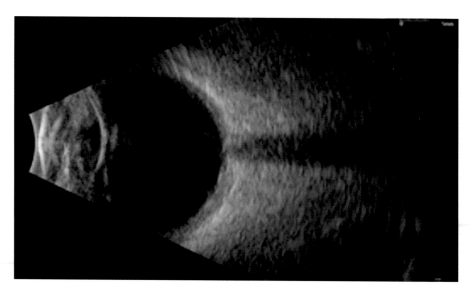

Figure 19.2 B scan of a normal globe: the hyperreflective structures at the left of the image represent the lens. The hyporeflective cavity is the vitreous. The optic nerve shadow can clearly be visualized as the horizontal hyporeflective strip at the right of the image.

CLINICAL CONTEXT TIPS

When would you use ocular ultrasound?

- Emergency clinic: to evaluate the status of the retina (tears / detachment) when there is no view through to the posterior segment (for example, due to cataract or vitreous haemorrhage) or for intraocular foreign body (this should only be undertaken by an experienced ocular sonographer when there is an open globe, in order not to cause extrusion of intraocular contents; see *Section 16.2.2*)
- Cataract clinic: to evaluate the status of the retina in dense cataracts with limited fundal view, especially if there is a relative afferent pupillary defect, a rapid or disproportionate decrease in vision, a history of retinal detachment, trauma or intravitreal injections or rubeosis
- Medical retina clinic: to evaluate retinal or choroidal mass lesions
- Other indications include looking for optic disc drusen (as a cause of pseudopapilloedema), papilloedema (measuring the optic nerve sheath diameter), choroidal detachments, and fluid in Tenon's space in posterior scleritis or orbital inflammation.

BOX 19.1: COMMON TERMS USED WHEN DESCRIBING B SCAN ULTRASOUND

- Brighter structures are described as hyperechoic; darker ones as hypoechoic
- Anechoic: no echo
- Attenuation: the sound waves have been absorbed (e.g. in tumours)
- Shadowing: the structure is so reflective that sound waves are not passing through it.
- Reverberation: sound waves are going back and forth (e.g. in a wooden foreign body)
- Gain: an amplifier function (higher gain gives 'brighter dots' but more unwanted signal; lower gain suppresses weaker signals and can improve resolution) – think of it like a dimmer switch
- Greyscale: can be thought of as sensitivity; a higher greyscale function displays more samples; a lower greyscale function displays fewer samples (can be used to improve resolution).

19.2 Performing an ocular ultrasound

1. Instil topical local anaesthetic.
2. On the ultrasound machine, enter details for a new patient.
3. Once the patient entry has been saved, select the eye (left/right) to be scanned.
4. Ensure the screen is visible to you: you should be focusing on the screen whilst

your probe is on the patient's eye.
5. Ensure the foot pedal is accessible to you.
6. Wind the ultrasound probe around your neck so that it doesn't fall.
7. Using your dominant hand, hold the probe like a pen and instil a small quantity of ultrasound gel.
8. Ultrasound can be performed on either closed or open eyes (for a better signal) once topical anaesthetic has been instilled. When starting, it may be most comfortable to perform this on closed eyes.
9. Place the probe directly on the eye, press the foot pedal to begin.
Different machines will be set up differently; however, there will be options to start and stop the recording of images, and to save still images from the scan with different foot pedal actions (e.g. double click, long click).
10. By convention, the probe is usually oriented with the marker upwards or nasally, depending on which cross-section you are imaging. For a transverse section, the patient looks in the direction you want to scan (similar to the fundal examination). The probe is then placed in the opposite direction to where you want to scan. In longitudinal sections, the probe points in the same direction as the patient is looking. Axial sections are taken with the eye in primary position. Orient yourself using the optic disc (black shadow; see *Figure 19.2*).
11. Use the different cross-sections to start to build a 3D image of the intraocular anomalies. Use a dynamic technique (asking the patient to look up, down, left and right) to gain a further idea of kinetic qualities of the tissues you are looking at.

19.3 Interpreting an ocular ultrasound

To describe a lesion, consider the following features:
- Topography: location, configuration and extension
- Reflectivity or echogenicity: its internal structure (a homogeneous appearance indicates no variation on the height of A scan spikes compared to heterogeneous appearance)
- Sound attenuation: is there any decrease in strength of echo within or posterior to the lesion? The denser the medium, the greater the absorption of sound
- Dynamic qualities: mobility of structures with or without eye movement
  - after-movement of tissues (more rapid if vitreous; less so if retinal)
  - intrinsic vascularity (spontaneous motion of echoes within a vascular lesion, suggestive of blood flow).

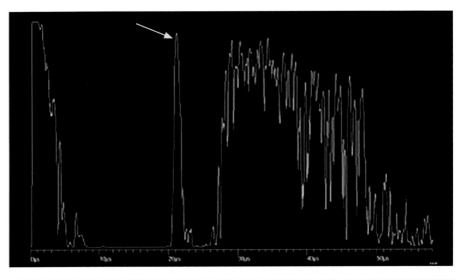

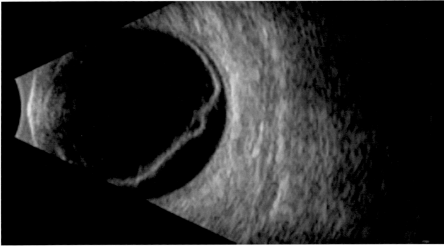

Figure 19.3 Retinal detachment: A scan (top) and B scan (bottom). The A scan shows a spike 100% of the height of the normal retinal spike (yellow arrow). The B scan shows a uniformly thick hyperechoic line which does not cross the optic nerve. Dynamic scanning would show a slow, undulating after-movement.

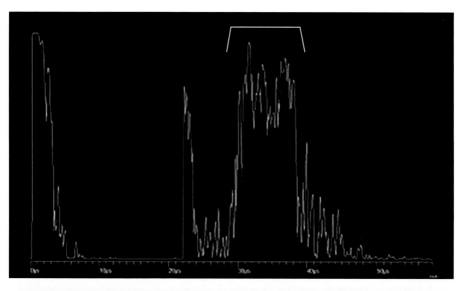

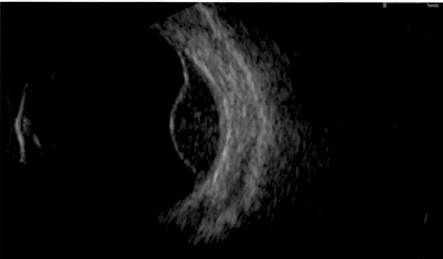

Figure 19.4 Choroidal melanoma: A scan (top) and B scan (bottom). Note the echogenic collar-stud / mushroom-shaped well-defined mass with low–medium internal reflectivity. The multiple spikes (highlighted by the yellow bracket) on the A scan where the mass is, represent high internal vascularity.

Chapter 20
Fundus fluorescein angiography

20.1 What is fundus fluorescein angiography and why do we use it?

Fundus fluorescein angiography (FFA) is an invasive diagnostic procedure used to assess the function and integrity of the choroidal and retinal circulation with an intravenous injection of sodium fluorescein.

20.1.1 How does it work?

FFA uses the fluorescent properties of the water-soluble dye sodium fluorescein to produce images of the retinal and choroidal vasculature. A custom-built camera is used to take a series of rapid sequence photographs once the sodium fluorescein has been administered into a vein via a cannula. This camera emits blue light (wavelength 465–490nm via the passage of white light through an excitation filter) that excites the sodium fluorescein molecules in the retinal vasculature. The sodium fluorescein then emits green light at a longer wavelength (520–530nm), which is captured by the barrier filter of the same fundus camera and converted to a digital image.

20.1.2 Indications

FFA can be useful in the diagnosis and management of the following diseases:
- Chorioretinal vascular disease
  - diabetic retinopathy (neovascularization, capillary non-perfusion and ischaemia)
  - retinal vein occlusion (neovascularization and ischaemia)
  - neovascular age-related macular degeneration (abnormal new choroidal blood vessel networks)
- Inherited retinal diseases (e.g. Stargardt's disease, Best's disease)
- Posterior uveitis and vasculitis
- Central serous retinopathy.

20.2 Performing an FFA

1. Preparation of the patient and obtaining informed consent:
   - *Table 20.1* illustrates the relative contraindications and side-effects of FFA for use when consenting the patient
   - The clinical room where the FFA is performed must have resuscitation and anaphylaxis medications present, readily available and functional
   - Baseline observations such as blood pressure, pulse and oxygen saturation must be performed
   - Cannulation must be completed for intravenous administration of the sodium fluorescein
   - Pupil dilation is required.

2. Patient is seated at the dedicated fundus camera, and a series of colour and red-free images are taken of each eye.
3. 5ml of 10% sodium fluorescein is injected as a bolus (over the course of a few seconds), whilst the photographer takes a series of images from both eyes for the next 5–10 minutes.
4. Late phase images are then taken at 20 minutes.
5. Once all images are obtained, the patient is directed back to the waiting room for observation for an hour to assess for any late allergic or anaphylactic response.

CLINICAL CONTEXT TIPS

How to fill out a request for FFA
When informing the photographer of the need for FFA, ensure to specify the **index eye**, which is the eye for which early images **must** be captured first due to more pronounced presence of pathology.

Table 20.1 Side-effects of FFA

Mild (common)	Moderate	Severe (rare)
Orange discolouration of skin and urine (24–48h)	Pyrexia	Anaphylaxis
	Urticaria	Bronchospasm
Transient nausea	Thrombophlebitis	Cardiac arrest
Vomiting	Syncope	Death (1 in 200 000)
Pruritus		
Extravasation of dye at injection site		
Relative contraindications: pregnancy		
Absolute contraindications: history of allergic hypersensitivity to fluorescein		

20.3 Phases of FFA

When 10% or 20% sodium fluorescein contrast dye is injected into the patient, it travels from the venous to the arterial circulation via the heart. From the heart the dye travels to the short posterior ciliary arteries to fill the choroidal vasculature. The retinal arteries are then filled a few seconds later, followed by the arterioles, capillaries and venous circulation. *Table 20.2* illustrates the different phases of FFA.

Table 20.2 Phases of FFA

Time	Phase	Anatomical correlation
10–15 seconds after injection	Choroidal	Dye arrives at the short ciliary arteries, followed by choroidal filling (*Figure 20.1A*) Cilioretinal vessel filling Prelaminar optic disc capillary filling
1–3 second(s) after choroidal phase	Arterial	Central retinal artery and arterial circulation filling (*Figure 20.1B*)
1–2 second(s) after arterial phase	Arteriovenous	Early: retinal arterioles and capillaries filling Late: laminar venous filling (where the walls of veins are filled first and the centre of the vein remains dark) (*Figure 20.1C*)
30 seconds (time after injection)	Venous	Total vein diameter filling (*Figure 20.1D*)
30 seconds to 10 minutes (time after injection)	Late phase/ recirculation	Dye no longer in the retinal vessels Staining of optic disc, Bruch's membrane, choroid and sclera

20.4 Interpretation of FFA

Simplistically, FFA images are interpreted in terms of areas of hyperfluorescence or hypofluorescence (*Figure 20.2*). The images obtained must be assessed in sequence of the phases discussed in the previous section.

20.4.1 Hyperfluorescence

There are five processes that cause hyperfluorescence on an FFA. The following is a summary of these processes, and how they are distinguishable from each other by differences in the area of hyperfluorescence (does it remain the same or enlarge over time?) and the border of hyperfluorescence (is it distinct or indistinct?), and in some cases, whether the intensity of the hyperfluorescence increases over time:

1. Leaking (early hyperfluorescence):
   - Loss of integrity of a vessel (e.g. choroidal neovascular membrane or neovascularization in retinal vascular occlusion)
   - Area: enlarges over time
   - Border: indistinct.
2. Pooling (early hyperfluorescence):
   - Gradual filling of fluid-filled space (e.g. in a serous pigment epithelial detachment)
   - Area: enlarges over time
   - Border: distinct.

3. Window defect (early hyperfluorescence):
   - Defect in the retinal pigment epithelium causing transillumination of choroidal hyperfluorescence (e.g. retinal pigment epithelium atrophy / loss)
   - Area, border and brightness of hyperfluorescence remains static over time.
4. Staining (late hyperfluorescence):
   - Accumulation of fluorescein dye (e.g. optic disc and drusen)
   - Area: remains static over time
   - Intensity: increases over time.
5. Autofluorescence (*Figure 20.3*):
   - Seen before injection of sodium fluorescein
   - Normally seen with drusen.

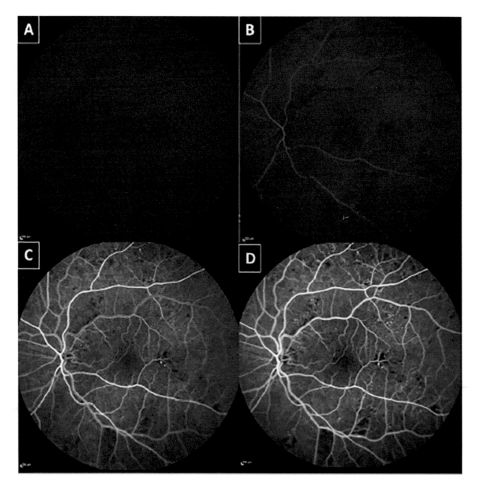

Figure 20.1 Phases of FFA: (A) choroidal; (B) arterial; (C) arteriovenous; (D) venous.

20.4.2 Hypofluorescence

When describing the pathology behind hypofluorescence, there are two main processes:

1. Transmission defect:
   - Fluorescein transmission is blocked
   - Blockage can be caused by blood, pigment, lipid and lipofuscin
   - Levels of blockage include preretinal (blocks both retinal and choroidal circulations), intraretinal (blocks capillary circulation but large retinal vessels can be visualized) and subretinal (blocks choroidal circulation).
2. Vascular filling defect:
   - Fluorescein transmission is blocked by non-perfusion of retinal vasculature.

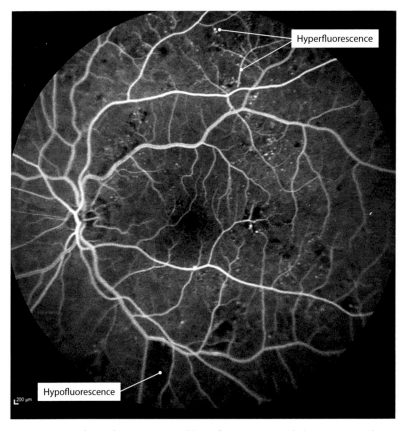

Figure 20.2 FFA hyperfluorescence and hypofluorescence in diabetic retinopathy.

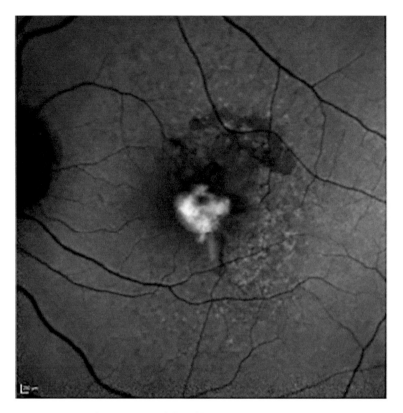

Figure 20.3 Autofluorescence exhibited by drusen at the macula.

Chapter 21
Systemic inflammation

There are both infectious and non-infectious causes of systemic inflammation, and ocular manifestations of systemic inflammation are variable. This chapter discusses the manifestations of non-infectious systemic inflammation, while *Chapter 22* covers the ocular manifestations of systemic infection.

Systemic inflammatory disorders can affect both the anterior and posterior segment of the eyes. Dry eye (*Section 9.2*), conjunctivitis (*Section 9.3.1*), keratitis (*Section 9.5.3*), uveitis (*Section 10.2*) and optic neuritis (*Section 14.5*) can all occur due to systemic inflammation. *Table 21.1* provides an A–Z guide of key systemic inflammatory conditions, their key clinical features and ocular manifestations. It allows clinicians to decipher clues when suspecting certain inflammatory conditions, and gives information on the special tests that can be performed to aid diagnosis. The key is to recognize the association of eye complaints with these conditions, and the importance of referring the patient to your local ophthalmology service for a comprehensive eye examination. Collaboration with rheumatology is also crucial, as they can guide investigation and management, particularly that of immunosuppressive treatment. Any patient with these conditions with subjective complaints of red eyes, blurred vision, loss of vision or diplopia, should be **referred urgently** to local eye services.

Table 21.1 Systemic inflammatory conditions and their ocular manifestations

Clinical features	Special tests	Ocular manifestations
Ankylosing spondylitis		
♂ > ♀ Age of onset: <45y Racial predilection: white patients (*"Do you suffer from back pain with stiffness mainly in the morning?"*)	HLA-B27	Anterior uveitis (see *Figure 10.1*)
Behçet's disease		
♂ = ♀ Age of onset: <30y Racial predilection: patients with Middle Eastern, Mediterranean and east Asian heritage Recurrent ulceration (*"Do you suffer from mouth or genital ulcers?"*)	HLA-B51	Anterior uveitis Posterior uveitis Retinal vasculitis

Clinical features	Special tests	Ocular manifestations
Dermatomyositis / polymyositis		
♀ > ♂ Age of onset: bimodal (5–15y and 45–65y) Racial predilection: none Proximal myopathy (*"Are you able to climb the stairs or comb your hair?"*) Rash (*"Do you have any purple rashes on your hands or on your nail cuticles?"*) Fever Weight loss	Elevated creatine kinase Antinuclear antibody (ANA) Anti-Mi-2 antibodies Anti-Jo-1 antibodies	Periorbital purple rash with oedema
Giant cell arteritis (GCA)		
♀ > ♂ Age of onset: >65y Racial predilection: more commonly reported in White patients, but is seen in other patient groups New-onset headache (see *Section 14.4*) Pain on chewing Transient loss of vision	ESR CRP Doppler of temporal arteries Temporal artery biopsy	Loss of vision Diplopia Central retinal artery occlusion (see *Figure 12.7*)
Granulomatosis with polyangiitis (GPA)		
♂ = ♀ Age of onset: 40–50y Racial predilection: more commonly reported in White patients, but is seen in other patient groups Unexplained fatigue and fever Nasal symptoms (*"Have you had a blocked nose recently?"* or *"Have you been having lots of nosebleeds?"*) Chronic ear infections Cough / chest pain	Anti-neutrophil cytoplasmic antibody (ANCA)	Peripheral ulcerative keratitis (see *Figure 9.8*) Scleritis (see *Figure 9.12*)

Table 21.1 *cont'd*

Clinical features	Special tests	Ocular manifestations
Inflammatory bowel disease (IBD)		
♂ = ♀ Age of onset: <30y Racial predilection: more commonly reported in White patients, but is seen in other patient groups Crohn's: can affect mouth (ulcers) to anus (diarrhoea) Ulcerative colitis: bloody diarrhoea Weight loss Iron-deficiency anemia (*"Have you had any changes to your bowel habit? Do you have increased fatigue or loss of appetite?"*)	ESR CRP Faecal calprotectin Colonoscopy	Conjunctivitis Episcleritis Anterior uveitis
Juvenile idiopathic arthritis (JIA)		
♀ > ♂ Age of onset: <16y Racial predilection: none Any child with chronic joint pain and swelling, and fatigue	ESR CRP ANA HLA-B27 Anti-cyclic citrullinated peptide antibodies (anti-CCP) Rheumatoid factor (RF)	Children diagnosed with JIA must be screened for uveitis within 6 weeks of diagnosis

Clinical features	Special tests	Ocular manifestations
Multiple sclerosis (MS)		
♀ > ♂ Age of onset: 20–40y (but can occur at any age) Racial predilection: none Optic neuritis symptoms (*"Do you have pain on eye movement and is your vision reduced?"*) Incontinence (*"Do you have any bowel or bladder problems?"*) Muscle weakness Charcot triad: ataxia, dysarthria and tremor Uhthoff's phenomenon: symptoms get worse in hot temperatures Lhermitte's sign: electrical sensation running down the back when the neck is flexed	MRI brain looking for hyperintense periventricular white matter lesions Oligoclonal bands in cerebrospinal fluid (CSF) from lumbar puncture If there is a more aggressive clinical course suggestive of neuromyelitis optica do blood tests for anti-aquaporin 4 antibodies	Intermediate uveitis Diplopia and nystagmus secondary to internuclear ophthalmoplegia (limitation of ipsilateral adduction) Optic neuritis
Myasthenia gravis (MG)		
♂ = ♀ Age of onset: any Racial predilection: none Limb weakness (*"Do you find it difficult getting yourself dressed or climbing stairs?"*) Ptosis (*"Do your eyelids droop more towards the end of the day?"*) Diplopia Dysphagia (*"Do you have issues swallowing?"*) Dysarthria (*"Do you ever find yourself slurring your words?"*) Dyspnoea (*"Do you find yourself being short of breath?"*)	Acetylcholine receptor antibodies Anti-MuSK	Variable ptosis Ophthalmoplegia causing diplopia

Table 21.1 *cont'd*

Clinical features	Special tests	Ocular manifestations
Polyarteritis nodosa (PAN)		
♂ > ♀ Age of onset: >50y Racial predilection: none Unexplained fever Skin ulcers Myalgia (*"Have you been having increasing muscle soreness recently?"*) Unexplained abdominal pain Unexplained hypertension	Negative ANCA Test for hepatitis B and C, and HIV	Ulcerative keratitis Scleritis
Psoriatic arthritis		
♂ = ♀ Age of onset: 35–55 Racial predilection: more commonly reported in White patients, but is seen in other patient groups Plaque-like skin rash (*"Do you have any rashes on your knees, elbows or scalp?"*) Joint pain (*"Do you have any swelling or pains in your joints?"*) Nail changes (*"Have you noticed any dents in your nails?"*)	HLA-B27	Conjunctivitis Dry eyes Keratitis Anterior uveitis
Reactive arthritis		
♂ = ♀ Age of onset: 20–40y Racial predilection: White patients GI symptoms Genito-urinary symptoms Joint pain and swelling (*"Have you been having diarrhoea symptoms, pain on urinating, genital discharge, or joint pain?"*)	Genito-urinary symptoms: test for chlamydia GI symptoms: test for *Campylobacter*, *Clostridioides difficile*, *Escherichia coli*, *Salmonella*, *Shigella*, *Yersinia*	Conjunctivitis Anterior uveitis

Clinical features	Special tests	Ocular manifestations
Rheumatoid arthritis (RA)		
♀ > ♂ Age of onset: any age but most likely with increasing age Racial predilection: more commonly reported in White patients, but is seen in other patient groups Joint pain and swelling (*"Do you have pain and stiffness in your joints, worse in the morning or after a period of inactivity?"*)	ESR CRP RF Anti-CCP antibodies	Dry eye Anterior uveitis Scleritis (see *Figure 9.12*)
Sarcoidosis		
♀ = ♂ Age of onset: 25–45y Racial predilection: Black patients Persistent dry cough (*"Have you had a cough lasting for more than 3 weeks? Is it dry or producing mucus?"*) Swollen lymph nodes (*"Do you have any swellings in your neck?"*) Erythema nodosum (*"Have you had any sore red bumps on your shins or ankles?"*)	Elevated ACE Chest X-ray (*hilar lymphadenopathy*) High resolution chest CT (*interstitial lung disease*)	Anterior and posterior uveitis ('candle wax retinitis')
Sjögren's syndrome		
♀ > ♂ Age of onset: 40–60y Racial predilection: none Dry mouth (*"Do you have difficulty speaking and swallowing?"*)	Anti-Ro antibodies Anti-La antibodies	Dry eye
Systemic sclerosis		
♀ > ♂ Age of onset: 40–50y Racial predilection: none Raynaud's phenomenon (*"Do your fingers go blue then white in cold weather?"*) Dysphagia (*"Do you have problems swallowing?"*)	Anti-topoisomerase 1 Anti-centromere antibody (ACA)	Tight periorbital skin

Table 21.1 *cont'd*

Clinical features	Special tests	Ocular manifestations
Systemic lupus erythematosus (SLE)		
♀ > ♂ Age of onset: 15–44y Racial predilection: Black and Chinese patients Butterfly rash (*"Do you have a facial rash or any joint pain or swelling?"*) Unexplained fever Joint and muscle ache Hair loss Sunlight sensitivity	ANA SLE-specific: anti-dsDNA or anti-Smith antibodies	Cranial nerve palsy III, IV and VI (see *Section 14.6.2*) Discoid lupus of the eyelids Dry eye Retinal vasculitis Scleritis Optic neuritis
Thyroid eye disease (TED)		
♀ > ♂ Age of onset: 30–50y Racial predilection: none Symptoms of overactive thyroid (*heat sensitivity, palpitations, unexplained weight loss, insomnia*) or underactive thyroid (*cold sensitivity, fatigue, unintentional weight gain, constipation, muscle aches*) Previous diagnosis of dysthyroid disease	TSH T_4 Thyroid peroxidase	Diplopia Dry eye Proptosis (see *Section 7.4.3*)

Chapter 22
Systemic infection

22.1 Introduction

Like systemic inflammation, systemic infection disease can cause different ocular manifestations. Sometimes ophthalmic signs may be the first (or only) clinical evidence of infection and timely work-up can be crucial in identifying and treating the underlying condition. Systemic infective conditions with ocular manifestations are less common but it is important to be aware of them.

In the following, we will work through each 'layer' of the eye and explore how systemic infection can affect each one, and then describe how to work patients up appropriately.

22.2 Conjunctivitis

We have already discussed the basics of bacterial, viral and allergic conjunctivitis in *Section 9.3.1.* Atypical conjunctivitis that is refractory to usual management, or a suspicious sexual history, should raise alarm bells for sexually transmitted disease.

History
Ask about:
- Onset
- Duration
- Preceding coryzal or viral illness
- Sexual history
- Systems review of genito-urinary symptoms (pain on passing urine, pelvic or testicular pain, discharge)
- Exposure to pets (cat scratch).

Examination
- Gonococcal
  - severe yellow–white purulent discharge
  - papillary tarsal conjunctival reaction
- Chlamydia
  - subacute eyelid swelling
  - mucopurulent discharge
  - follicular tarsal conjunctival reaction
- *Bartonella*
  - unilateral follicular conjunctivitis
  - dilated fundus exam should be performed to check for neuro-retinitis (optic disc swelling with macular star-shaped exudate deposition)
- Look for pseudomembranes on lid eversion and rule out consequent keratopathy
- Include checking for regional lymphadenopathy.

Investigations
- Urgent conjunctival swabs for microscopy, culture and sensitivity and chlamydia PCR
- *Bartonella* serology.

Management
In accordance with local protocol, but typically involves:
- Topical antibiotics
  - gonorrhoea: 2-hourly topical quinolone antibiotic drops and saline irrigation
  - chlamydia: 6-hourly topical erythromycin antibiotic drops / ointment
  - *Bartonella*: depends on local policy and ranges from supportive to topical antibiotic eye drops to systemic antibiotics
  - removal of pseudomembranes at the slit lamp
- Referral to the sexual health clinic for systemic treatment, follow-up and contact tracing
- Liaison with the paediatric safeguarding team for any suspected cases in children.

22.3 Keratitis

The corneal infections discussed in *Section 9.4* tend to be more severe in immunocompromised patients (e.g. HIV patients), but certain corneal presentations can in themselves raise suspicion for an underlying systemic infection.

Interstitial keratitis presents as a salmon-pink lesion with a lighter border with surrounding corneal haze and corneal vascularization in the affected sector. It represents an immune-mediated antigen-triggered type 4 hypersensitivity reaction, with non-suppurative stromal inflammation, without epithelial or endothelial involvement. Active ulcerative keratitis should be ruled out.

Infectious causes of interstitial keratitis include syphilis, herpes and tuberculosis. Approximately 90% of cases are due to congenital syphilis for which a pre- and postnatal history should be obtained (failure to thrive, deafness, birth history and maternal history for syphilis).

Examination
- See *Section 9.4* for clinical findings in keratitis
- Look for **Hutchinson's triad** (peg teeth, deafness and interstitial keratitis) if suspicious for syphilis
- On dilated fundoscopy look for:
  - posterior uveitis (placoid – *think syphilis*; serpiginous – *think tuberculosis*)
  - retinitis (*think herpetic disease*; see *Figure 22.2*).

Investigations
- Corneal scrapings can be taken if there is suspicion of active ocular surface infection
- Syphilis serology
- QuantiFERON-Gold (*think tuberculosis*)
- Viral serology (*think herpetic disease*).

Management
- Topical steroids: to manage local immune-mediated inflammation, to reduce pain and scarring risk
- Collaboration with the infectious disease team is important to treating the underlying cause
- Surgery with optical keratoplasty can be considered but there remains a risk of rejection.

22.4 Scleritis

Scleritis (discussed in *Section 9.8*) can cause a diffusely red eye associated with deep ache and globe tenderness. This is in comparison to episcleritis, a self-limiting condition with sectoral redness and irritation.

Investigations
Serology and QuantiFERON-Gold will guide treatment for the underlying disease. Treatment should be initiated in collaboration with the infectious disease team.

Management
Most scleritis is non-infective immune-related disease (see *Chapter 21*) and can be treated with topical and/or oral steroids, NSAIDs and treating the underlying systemic inflammation. However, scleritis can also be associated with systemic infection such as syphilis, Lyme disease, tuberculosis and varicella zoster.

22.5 Uveitis

Uveitis has been discussed in *Section 10.2*. It can be classified anatomically (anterior, intermediate, posterior or panuveitis) or by aetiology (infectious, non-infectious and masquerade: non-neoplastic and neoplastic).

The aetiology of infectious uveitis includes:
- Bacterial: e.g. syphilis, tuberculosis, Lyme disease
- Viral: e.g. herpes zoster, herpes simplex, cytomegalovirus
- Fungal: e.g. candida
- Other: e.g. toxoplasmosis, *Toxocara*.

These can result in typical ocular findings of:
- Painful, red eye with reduced vision and photophobia
- Circumlimbal injection with anterior chamber activity
- Iris changes
- Posterior segment inflammation
- Vitritis
- Chorio-retinal lesions
- Vasculitis
- Rarely, optic neuritis or cranial nerve palsies.

Characteristic ocular features of each of the main infection types are described in *Table 22.1*.

Table 22.1 Typical ophthalmic features of some infectious uveitides

Infection	Type of uveitis	Characteristic features
Syphilis	Unilateral / bilateral Granulomatous / non-granulomatous Anterior / posterior / panuveitis	Papillary conjunctivitis Interstitial keratitis (congenital infection) Iris roseola Placoid fundal lesions (*Figure 22.1*)
Tuberculosis	Unilateral / bilateral Caseating granulomatous / non-granulomatous Anterior / posterior (more common – choroidal involvement)	Lid tubercle Conjunctival phlycten Broad posterior synechiae Iris granulomas Choroidal lesions: tuberculomas, serpiginous lesions, vasculitis, periphlebitis
Lyme disease	Unilateral / bilateral Granulomatous Anterior (more common) / intermediate / posterior	Erythema multiforme Follicular conjunctivitis Episcleritis Interstitial keratitis Chorioretinal plaques Vasculitis Cranial nerve palsies (especially facial nerve)
Herpetic (varicella zoster virus (VZV) and herpes simplex virus (HSV))	Unilateral, non-granulomatous, anterior If associated with acute retinal necrosis (ARN): unilateral granulomatous panuveitis – can progress to bilateral If associated with progressive outer retinal necrosis (PORN): unilateral / bilateral, more posterior involvement	ARN (*Figure 22.2*): pain, vitritis, peripheral necrotizing retinitis, vasculitis, retinal detachment, optic neuropathy PORN: coalescing outer retinal necrosis with central involvement

Infection	Type of uveitis	Characteristic features
Cytomegalovirus	Unilateral, can progress to bilateral Non-granulomatous Posterior	Minimal anterior chamber inflammation Haemorrhagic / granular retinitis ('pizza pie' appearance) 'Frosted branch' angiitis (perivascular retinitis)
Candida	Unilateral / bilateral Anterior / intermediate / posterior (more common)	Vitritis Multifocal chorioretinitis with 'string of pearls' appearance
Toxoplasma	Unilateral / bilateral Necrotizing granulomatous Anterior / posterior (more common)	Moderate anterior uveitis Vitritis with retinochoroiditis (choroidal lesions; see *Figure 22.3*) – 'headlight in the fog' appearance Previous pigmented scars Retinal vasculitis
Toxocara	Unilateral Non-granulomatous Anterior / posterior (more common)	Diffuse unilateral chronic non-granulomatous endophthalmitis Posterior pole granuloma Peripheral granuloma (retinal traction with fibrous bands)

A full history and systems review should be undertaken to assess for infection exposure and systemic symptoms relating to the primary infection (e.g. chest pain, cough, dyspnoea, genito-urinary symptoms, rashes, neurological symptoms, fevers). If clinical suspicion remains, investigations can include QuantiFERON-Gold and serology screening. Aqueous and vitreous PCR sampling can also be undertaken for infective causes (and to rule out neoplasm). Patients with infectious uveitis benefit from being under the care of a uveitis specialist for more tailored management and follow-up.

22.6 Endophthalmitis

Endophthalmitis is a post-operative complication of ocular surgery (exogenous aetiology; see *Section 11.5*). However, endophthalmitis can also be endogenous from haematological infective spread (pathogens reaching the eye via the bloodstream). This is rare, but can be devastating to visual function. The causes are mostly bacterial or fungal, though rarely can be viral or parasitic.

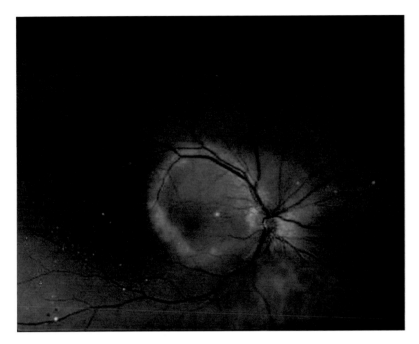

Figure 22.1 Part of a wide-field fundus photograph showing placoid lesions, as seen in ocular syphilis.

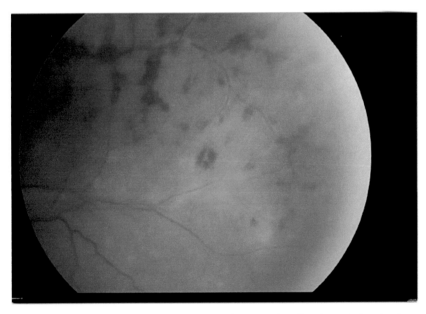

Figure 22.2 Colour fundus photo of acute retinal necrosis (ARN) in the peripheral retina secondary to herpetic eye disease. Note the haemorrhagic changes around the retinal vessels with occlusive retinal arteriolitis (suggestive of retinal necrosis).

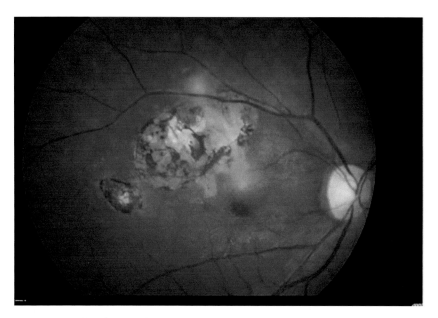

Figure 22.3 Colour fundus photograph of the right eye affected by toxoplasmosis. Note the discrete pigmented chorioretinal macular lesions (*Toxoplasma* scars) with a fluffy white lesion emerging at the superior arcade indicating active infection.

History

Ask about risk factors:
- Recent invasive procedures
- Recent systemic infection (primary cause from liver / respiratory / neurological)
- Immunocompromised
- Intravenous drug use
- Indwelling catheters.

Examination

There is a spectrum of presentation, from insidious onset, with cases picked up on screening, to red, painful eyes with vision loss. Examination typically reveals anterior and posterior segment inflammation (choroidal infiltrates with overlying vitritis) and may need ocular ultrasound to facilitate posterior segment examination if there is no fundal view. Screening for candida endogenous endophthalmitis is performed for intensive care patients with positive blood / line cultures for candida (in accordance with local hospital policy).

Investigation

Diagnostic work-up should include:
- Ocular fluid sampling for stain, culture and PCR
- Blood tests including bacterial and fungal cultures, and serology for systemic infection (e.g. HIV, *Toxoplasma*, hepatitis, syphilis, QuantiFERON-Gold, Lyme disease).

Depending on the clinical picture, also include:

- Urine cultures
- CSF cultures
- Brain, chest, liver and heart imaging (looking for abscesses and valvular vegetations).

Management

This should be in accordance with local policy and include:

- Intravitreal tap and injection of intravitreal antibiotics with consideration of vitrectomy, as per the exogenous endophthalmitis protocol (see *Section 11.5*)
- Removal of the inciting cause (e.g. catheter or line)
- Systemic antimicrobial therapy in collaboration with the medical and microbiology team.

22.7 Retinal signs of systemic infection

There are specific retinal signs that can point towards certain diagnoses:

- Macular stars: in neuroretinitis, these represent hard exudates arranged in a radial pattern due to the alignment of fibres in the outer plexiform layer. Macular stars can be idiopathic, inflammatory, or a sign of malignant hypertension (so be sure to check BP), but they can also have an infective aetiology, specifically *Bartonella* (see *Section 22.2*), syphilis, *Toxoplasma* and *Toxocara*. Management includes serology testing and treatment of the underlying cause.
- Roth spots: white-centred retinal haemorrhages (which represent retinal capillary rupture and platelets sticking to damaged endothelium with fibrin-platelet thrombi; *Figure 22.4*). They can be a sign of haematological disease, e.g. leukaemia, diabetic retinopathy or trauma, but can also represent infective aetiology such as bacterial endocarditis or HIV. If seen, ask about immunocompromise and recent invasive procedures (including dental and endoscopic prostate procedures). Endocarditis is rare but fatal if untreated, and you may be the first to pick it up.
- Vasculitis, haemorrhagic or necrotizing retinitis (see *Figure 22.2*): if infective, may represent acute retinal necrosis and peripheral outer retinal necrosis (the most common aetiologic agents being VZV, HSV and cytomegalovirus associated with HIV). Retinitis can appear as well-demarcated spreading whitened areas of retina with scalloped edges (necrotizing), haemorrhages (haemorrhagic), non-perfused/leaking retinal vessels (vasculitis), with or without vitreal or anterior segment inflammation. Risk factors for immunocompromise should be noted. Investigations include ocular fluid sampling with viral PCR and systemic infection work-up. Co-infection with syphilis, *Toxoplasma* or tuberculosis should be ruled out. Management includes treating the underlying systemic condition and any anterior uveitis, as well as intravitreal antivirals. Systemic treatment may be lifelong. Advanced cases require laser or surgical ocular intervention, though prognosis can be poor.

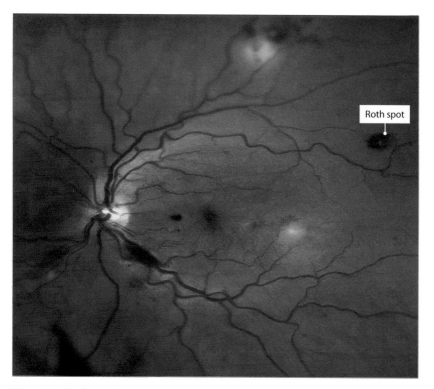

Figure 22.4 Roth spot in a patient with acute myeloid leukaemia.

Snellen chart for distance vision measurement

6/60	**E**	1	20/200
6/30	**F P**	2	20/100
6/20	**T O Z**	3	20/70
6/15	**L P E D**	4	20/50
6/12	**P E C F D**	5	20/40
6/9	**E D F C Z P**	6	20/30
6/7.5	**F E L O P Z D**	7	20/25
6/6	**D E F P O T E C**	8	20/20
6/5	L E F O D P C T	9	
	F D P L T C E O	10	
	P E Z O L C F T D	11	

Hold 1 metre away from patient

Jaeger near vision chart

Jaeger Chart

No. 1
.37 M

IIn the second century of the Christian aera, the empire of Rome comprehended the fairest part of the earth, and the most civilized portion of mankind. The frontiers of that extensive monarchy were guarded by ancient renown and disciplined valour. The gentle, but powerful, influence of laws and manners had gradually cemented the union of the provinces. Their peaceful inhabitants enjoyed and abused the advantages of wealth

No. 2
.50 M

and luxury. The image of a free constitution was preserved with decent reverence. The Roman senate appeared to possess the sovereign authority, and devolved on the emperors all the executive powers of government. During a happy period of more than fourscore years, the public administration was conducted by the virtue and abilities of Nerva, Trajan,

No. 3
.62 M

Hadrian, and the two Antonines. It is the design of this and of the two succeeding chapters, to describe the prosperous condition of their empire; and afterwards, from the death of Marcus Antoninus, to deduce the most important circumstances of its decline and fall: a revolution which will ever be remembered, and is still felt by the nations of the earth.

No. 4
.75 M

The principal conquests of the Romans were achieved under the republic; and the emperors, for the most part, were satisfied with preserving those dominions which had been acquired by the policy of the senate, the active emulation of the consuls, and the martial enthusiasm of the people. The seven first centuries were filled with a rapid succession of triumphs;

No. 5
1.00 M

but it was reserved for Augustus to relinquish the ambitious design of subduing the whole earth, and to introduce a spirit of moderation into the public councils. Inclined to peace by his temper and situation, it was easy for him to discover that

No. 6
1.25 M

that Rome, in her present exalted situation, had much less to hope than to fear from the chance of arms; and that, in the prosecution of remote wars, the undertaking became every day more difficult, the event more doubtful, and the possession more precarious and less beneficial.

No. 7
1.50 M

The experience of Augustus added weight to these salutary reflections, and effectually convinced him that, by the prudent vigour of his counsels, it would be easy to secure every concession which the safety or the dignity of Rome

No. 8
1.75 M

might require from the most formidable barbarians. Instead of exposing his person and his legions to the arrows of the Parthians, he obtained, by an honorable

No. 9
2.00 M

treaty, the restitution of the standards and prisoners which had been taken in the defeat of Crassus. His generals, in the early part of his reign,

No.10
2.25 M

attempted the reduction of Aethiopia and Arabia Felix. They marched near a thousand miles to the south of the tropic; but the heat of the

No. 11
2.50 M

the climate soon repelled the invaders and protected the unwarlike natives of those sequestered regions.

Index

Bold indicates main entry